1001 Questions about Radiologic Technology

Volume 4

1001 Questions about Radiologic Technology

Volume 4

Roy Bell, B.A., B.S. (in Ed.), FASRT

Director
Community Hospital School of Radiologic Technology
Salem, Ohio

University Park Press • Baltimore

University Park Press
International Publishers in Medicine and Human Services
300 North Charles Street
Baltimore, Maryland 21201

Sponsoring editor: Ruby Richardson
Production editor: Michael Treadway
Cover design by: Caliber Design Planning, Inc.

Typeset by: Ampersand Publishers Services, Inc.
Manufactured in the United States of America by: Halliday Lithograph

Library of Congress Cataloging in Publication Data
(Revised for vol. 4)

Bell, Roy, 1930–
    1001 questions about radiologic technology.

    Includes bibliographies.
    1. Radiography, Medical—Examinations, questions, etc.   2. Medical technology—
Examinations, questions, etc.
I. Title.   [DNLM: 1. Technology, Radiologic—Examination questions. WN 18 058]
RC78.B393   616.07' 57' 076   80–137150
ISBN 0-8391-2086-9

To Marilyn, Rufena, Gayle, Cheryl and Bill
who paved the way for all the rest

Contents

Preface

The wide acceptance of the first three volumes in this series has prompted the writing of Volume 4. This is a companion volume to Volumes 1, 2, and 3, and not a substitute or replacement for them. The previously unpublished questions have been completely referenced in order to facilitate the review process. The references are identified by number as they are listed at the back of the book; this number is followed by the first page number in the reference where the answer can be found. Use of these references will make the review process more meaningful and more valuable to the student.

This volume and the previous volumes have been written for students who are preparing to take the ARRT examination in Radiography. Many of the questions, however, are directly applicable to the certifying examinations in Nuclear Medicine Technology, Radiation Therapy Technology, and Diagnostic Medical Sonography. This book may also serve as a valuable self-assessment tool for the practicing radiologic technologist. Instructors may also wish to use this volume, or the entire series, as the basis for review sessions, and their comments or suggestions are welcome.

Section 1

Principles of Radiographic Exposure and Processing

1. A filter is placed at the tube port to
   A. Decrease the production of scattered radiation
   B. Decrease the production of secondary radiation
   C. Reduce the number of unnecessary photons reaching the patient's body
   D. Make the x-ray beam less energetic
   E. Make the x-ray beam less homogeneous   5:229

2. The most effective device for preventing scattered radiation from reaching the film is the
   A. Filter
   B. Grid
   C. Collimator
   D. Cone
   E. Rare earth screen   10:46

3. When a radiographic image appears to be elongated, the primary factor to change is
   A. Screen speed
   B. Focal-film distance
   C. Object-film distance
   D. Target-object-film alignment
   E. Milliamperage   10:93

4. If the original MAS at a 40-inch focal-film distance is 12, and the focal-film distance is changed to 60 inches, the new MAS to maintain density is
   A. 7.2
   B. 11.9
   C. 19.3
   D. 27
   E. 34   4:103

$$\frac{I'}{I^2} = \left(\frac{D^2}{D_1}\right)^2 \qquad \frac{12\ mAS}{x} = \left(\frac{60\ cm}{40\ cm}\right)^2$$

$$12x = (1.5)^2$$
$$12x = 2.25$$
$$x = 12 \times 2.25$$
$$x = 27$$

5. Which of the following patient factors would be least valuable in determining correct radiographic exposure?
   A. Age
   B. Sex
   C. Height
   D. Body habitus
   E. Pathologic processes   4:81

6. The term body habitus refers to
   A. The chemical composition of body parts
   B. Maintenance of physiologic equilibrium
   C. Body posture
   D. Physique
   E. Muscle tone   4:74

7. An x-ray beam in which all of the photons have the same energy
    is said to be
    I.   Homogeneous
    II. Heterogeneous
    III. Monoenergetic
    IV. Polyenergetic
    A. I, III
    B. II, IV
    C. I, IV
    D. II, III
    E. I   4:65

8. Beam intensity has a direct influence on which of the following?
    I.   Radiographic density
    II. Radiographic sharpness
    III. Radiographic distortion
    A. I
    B. II
    C. III
    D. I, II
    E. I, II, III   4:60

9. If the radiographic image is not a true representation of the size
    or shape of the part, the effect is known as
    A. Divergence
    B. Diffraction
    C. Penumbra
    D. Distortion
    E. Superimposition   4:51

10. As an x-ray tube ages, its output is most likely to
    A. Fluctuate
    B. Increase
    C. Decrease
    D. Remain unchanged
    E. Completely stop   4:47

11. Poor film-screen contact can usually be identified by
    A. Generalized blurring of the image
    B. Localized blurring of the image
    C. Decreased density
    D. Increased density
    E. Increased contrast   4:39

12. Usually, a radiographic film that exhibits wide latitude will also
    exhibit
    A. Slow speed
    B. Fast speed
    C. Low contrast
    D. High contrast
    E. Increased resolution   4:21

13. Blue tint is added to the base of radiographic film to
    A. Decrease the parallax effect
    B. Increase radiographic density
    C. Improve radiographic contrast
    D. Increase resolution
    E. Refract the light from the illuminator   4:14

14. All of the following directly affect radiographic contrast except
    A. Processing
    B. Screen type and speed
    C. FFD
    D. Body density
    E. Kilovoltage   4:12

15. Radiographic density is dependent on which of the following?
    I.   Film speed
    II. Body thickness
    III. The amount of exposure
    A. I
    B. I, II
    C. I, II, III
    D. II, III
    E. III   4:5

16. Select the set of technical factors that will produce the greatest
    density.

	MA	Time in sec	KV	FFD in inches	Screen speed
A.	300	.60 /80	80	50	Par
B.	200	.50 /00	92	40	High
C.	400	.30 /00	92	60	Par
D.	500	.20 /00	80	30	Detail
E.	100	.20 0	80	50	Detail

                                                                 5:311

17. Select the missing factor that will produce the same radiographic
    density as the original factors.

         200 MA   400 MA
         0.5 sec   to   1 sec
         90 KVP   ____ KVP

    A. 45
    B. 50
    C. 65
    D. 70
    E. 85   5:306

18. Which type of effect is likely to occur at a kilovoltage range
    of 35 to 70 KVP?
    A. Complete penetration
    B. Photoelectric interaction
    C. Compton interaction
    D. Partial penetration
    E. Pair production   5:221

19. Reasons for manipulating kilovoltage settings for general radiography include
    - I.   To maintain proper contrast
    - II.   To assure adequate part penetration
    - III. To regulate radiographic density
    - A. I
    - B. I, II
    - C. I, II, III
    - D. II, III
    - E. III   5:193

20. Exposure time has a direct influence on which characteristic of the x-ray beam?
    - A. Intensity
    - B. Penetrating power
    - C. Quality
    - D. Quantity
    - E. Energy   5:127

21. All of the following are usually found in an intensifying screen except the
    - A. Abrasion layer
    - B. Active crystal layer
    - C. Refractive layer
    - D. Reflective layer
    - E. Plastic backing   5:78

22. An increase in KVP will produce which of the following?
    - I.   Increased beam efficiency
    - II.   Decreased patient dose
    - III. Decreased radiation fog
    - A. I
    - B. I, II
    - C. I, II, III
    - D. I, III
    - E. II   5:189

23. Changes which decrease the effects of penumbra include
    - I.   Decreased focal-film distance
    - II.   Decreased object-film distance
    - III. Decreased focal spot size
    - A. I
    - B. II
    - C. III
    - D. II, III
    - E. I, III   10:88

24. The number of gray tones that appear on a radiograph is controlled by
    - A. KVP
    - B. MAS
    - C. Filtration
    - D. Screen speed
    - E. Beam restriction   10:33

25. The formula for finding the new MAS for changes in FFD is

A. $\dfrac{\text{Original MAS X New FFD}^2}{\text{Old FFD}^2}$

B. $\dfrac{\text{Original MAS X Old FFD}^2}{\text{New FFD}^2}$

C. $\dfrac{\text{New FFD}^2 \text{ X Old FFD}^2}{\text{Original MAS}}$

D. $\dfrac{\text{Original MAS}}{\text{New FFD}^2} \text{ X Old FFD}^2$

E. $\dfrac{\text{Old FFD}^2}{\text{New FFD}^2} \text{ X Original MAS}$

4:103

26. In general, a body region of low subject contrast requires the use of
    A. Higher kilovoltage
    B. Lower kilovoltage
    C. A high ratio grid
    D. A low ratio grid
    E. A small focal spot   4:80

27. A kilovoltage setting of 120 is equivalent to _____ volt(s).
    A. 1/120
    B. 120
    C. 1200
    D. 12,000
    E. 120,000   4:73

28. Focal-film distance influences which of the following?
    I.   Radiographic density
    II. Image size
    III. Radiographic sharpness
    A. I, II
    B. I, III
    C. II, III
    D. I, II, III
    E. III   4:60

29. On which of the following does MA have the greatest effect?
    A. Part penetration
    B. Radiographic density
    C. Kinetic energy of the space charge
    D. Radiographic contrast
    E. Subject contrast   4:49

30. When the cathode filament is heated to the point that it glows, it is said to be
    A. Saturated
    B. Fluorescent
    C. Incandescent
    D. Luminescent
    E. Thermal   4:47

✓31. Quantum mottle would probably be most noticeable when
    A. Low KVP is used with slow speed screens
    B. Low MAS is used with slow speed screens
    C. High KVP is used with slow speed screens
    D. High MAS is used with slow speed screens
    E. High KVP is used with fast speed screens   4:39

✓32. If a radiographic film is developed without being exposed, its appearance will be
    A. Completely transparent
    B. Completely gray
    C. Clear, but not completely transparent
    D. Completely green
    E. Completely black   4:20

✓33. Which of the following best describes the effect of overdevelopment of a radiograph?
    A. Increased contrast and decreased density
    B. Increased contrast and increased density
    C. Decreased contrast and decreased density
    D. Decreased contrast and increased density
    E. Increased visibility of detail and decreased definition
                                                                              4:12

✓34. Effects of high developer temperature include
    I. Increased radiographic density
    II. Production of a shorter scale of contrast
    III. Increased radiographic contrast
    A. I
    B. II
    C. III
    D. I, II
    E. I, II, III   4:11

✓35. As subject contrast increases,
    A. Radiographic contrast is likely to decrease
    B. Radiographic contrast is likely to increase
    C. Radiographic density is likely to increase
    D. Radiographic definition is likely to increase
    E. Less kilovoltage is required for penetration of the part
                                                                              4:3

36. Select the set of technical factors that will produce the shortest
    scale of contrast.

	MA	Time in sec	KV	FFD in inches	Grid ratio
A.	100	.10	60	40	Nongrid
B.	300	.10	60	50	5:1
C.	200	.15	60	40	6:1
D.	400	.10	60	40	8:1
E.	300	.15	60	40	5:1

                                                          5:311

37. A 5:1 grid ratio is recommended for kilovoltage settings no
    greater than _____ KVP.
    A. 60
    B. 70
    C. 80
    D. 100
    E. 120   5:266

38. All of the following are reasons for a high degree of subject
    contrast in the chest region except
    A. A wide variation in tissue density
    B. A large amount of air
    C. A variety of tissues
    D. A large number of solid organs
    E. Lack of compactness of tissues   5:217

39. The amount of scattered radiation produced during a radiographic
    exposure is dependent on all of the following except
    A. Field size
    B. Focal spot size
    C. KVP level
    D. Thickness of tissue
    E. Density of tissue   5:191

40. All of the following terms belong to the group except
    A. Electrical pressure
    B. Kilovoltage
    C. Electrical imbalance
    D. Quality
    E. Resistance   5:174

41. Which of the following will result from a decrease in milliamper-
    age?
      I. Decreased contrast
     II. Decreased photon production
    III. Increased ionization of silver bromide crystals
    A. I
    B. II
    C. III
    D. I, II
    E. I, II, III   5:124

42. Functions of the recirculation system in a processor include
    I.   Maintenance of chemical strength
    II. Maintenance of temperature
    III. Conservation of silver
    A. I
    B. II
    C. III
    D. I, II
    E. I, II, III   5:67

43. A chest radiograph demonstrates an area of unsharpness in the
    left apex. The most likely cause is
    A. Variation of solution temperatures in the processor
    B. The use of excessive kilovoltage
    C. A stain on the front intensifying screen
    D. A stain on the rear intensifying screen
    E. Poor screen-film contact   4:117

44. The most important factor for minimizing involuntary motion is
    A. Immobilization
    B. Beam restriction
    C. Screen speed
    D. Exposure time
    E. Filtration   10:85

45. An original exposure time is 1/8 second at a focal-film distance
    of 36 inches. The exposure time needed to produce comparable
    density at a focal-film distance of 72 inches is _____ second.
    A. 1/32
    B. 1/16
    C. 1/4
    D. 1/2
    E. 1   4:103

46. Correct statements about the fluid content of the body include
    I.   It is greater than usual around a traumatized area
    II. It is less than usual around a traumatized area
    III. It is higher in young people
    IV. It is lower in young people
    A. I, III
    B. II, IV
    C. I, IV
    D. II, III
    E. II   4:82

47. All of the following are classified as basic body substances in
    the process of x-ray absorption and radiographic contrast <u>except</u>
    A. Bone
    B. Water
    C. Air
    D. Fat
    E. Skin   4:74

48. Which of the following body regions has the highest subject contrast?
    A. Neck
    B. Chest
    C. Abdomen
    D. Pelvis
    E. Hip   4:65

49. Which of the following best explains the inverse square law?
    A. The x-ray beam tends to diverge, causing intensity to increase.
    B. The x-ray beam tends to diverge, causing intensity to decrease.
    C. The x-ray beam tends to spread, causing definition to increase.
    D. The x-ray beam tends to spread, causing definition to decrease.
    E. The intensity of the x-ray beam and radiographic definition
       are inversely proportional to beam divergence.   4:60

50. If an original beam intensity is 5 MR at a FFD of 30 inches, the
    beam intensity at 60 inches will be _____ MR.
    A. 0.625
    B. 1.25
    C. 2.50
    D. 10
    E. 20   4:52

51. A major problem with automatic exposure control is
    A. Backup timing often interferes with the exposure
    B. It is inefficient when high KVP technique is used
    C. It is inefficient when high MAS technique is used
    D. It does not work well at long exposure times
    E. Positioning of the part is critical   4:47

52. The term that refers to the quantity of electrons moving from the
    cathode to the anode of the x-ray tube is
    A. Saturation current
    B. Space charge effect
    C. Milliamperage
    D. Kilovoltage
    E. Resistance   4:41

53. Chemical fog may occur under which of the following circumstances?
    I.   When unexposed crystals are reduced
    II. When the developer temperature is too high
    III. When the replenishment rate is too great
    A. I
    B. II
    C. III
    D. I, II
    E. I, II, III   4:22

54. Base fog is considered excessive if it goes beyond a density
    range of
    A. 0.002
    B. 0.003
    C. 0.02
    D. 0.03
    E. 0.2   4:14

55. As compared to the variable KVP method, the fixed KVP technique chart will
    I.   Produce more exposure latitude
    II. Decrease patient dose
    III. Provide a longer scale of contrast
    A. I
    B. I, II
    C. I, II, III
    D. II, III
    E. III   4:71

56. The H and D curve can determine which of the following?
    I.   Density
    II. Contrast
    III. Latitude
    A. I
    B. II
    C. III
    D. I, II
    E. I, II, III   4:5

Refer to the following technical factors for the next question.

	MA	Time in sec	KV	FFD in inches	Screen speed
I.	500	.25 125	80	55	Slow
II.	400	.15 60	90	40	Par
III.	200	.12 24	70	30	Slow
IV.	100	.20 20	80	60	Par

57. Rank these technical factors in order from greatest to least density.
    A. I, II, III, IV
    B. II, I, III, IV
    C. I, II, IV, III
    D. II, III, I, IV
    E. III, I, II, IV   5:311

58. Select the missing factor that will produce the same radiographic density as the original factors.

        5 MAS   _____ MAS
        80 KVP   to   80 KVP
        40" FFD   40" FFD
        Nongrid   6:1 grid
    A. 6
    B. 8
    C. 12
    D. 15
    E. 18   5:311

59. Scattered photons are produced by which of the following?
    I. Photoelectric interaction
    II. Compton interaction
    III. Unmodified interaction
    A. I
    B. II
    C. III
    D. I, II
    E. II, III   5:227

60. Body part thickness in cm x 2 + 30 KVP.
    This formula is used for establishing _____ KVP.
    A. Maximum
    B. Minimum
    C. Effective
    D. Average
    E. Base   5:193

61. When electrons are decelerated in the process of x-ray production,
    their kinetic energy is converted into
    I. Heat
    II. X-rays
    III. Gamma rays
    IV. Sound
    A. I, II
    B. I, II, III
    C. I, II, III, IV
    D. II, III, IV
    E. II   5:176

62. Exposure time has some influence on which of the following?
    I. Visibility of detail
    II. Radiographic density
    III. Sharpness of detail
    A. I
    B. I, II
    C. I, II, III
    D. II, III
    E. II   5:127

63. If 50 MAS and 60 KVP are the required technical factors for
    radiography with nonscreen technique, and the factors required
    for radiography with screen technique are 2.5 MAS and 60 KVP,
    the screen intensification factor is
    A. 0.05
    B. 2.5
    C. 20
    D. 25
    E. 125   5:85

64. Causes of unsafe safelighting include
    I.   Fading of the safelight filter
    II. Leaking of light from the safelight
    III. Bulb wattage greater than specified
    A. I
    B. I, II
    C. I, II, III
    D. II, III
    E. III   15:255

65. Causes of true distortion include
    I.   Improper alignment of the tube and the film
    II. Improper angulation of the tube
    III. Improper alignment of the part and the film
    A. I, II
    B. I, III
    C. I, II, III
    D. II, III
    E. III   10:83

66. In order to produce the greatest definition, the preferred screen
    speed is ____; in order to use the shortest exposure time, the
    preferred screen speed is ____; in order to attain the greatest
    density, the preferred screen speed is _____.
    A. High; detail; high
    B. Detail; high; high
    C. High; high; high
    D. Detail; detail; detail
    E. Par; detail; high   10:56

67. The chief reason for using a moving grid rather than a stationary
    grid is that the moving grid
    A. Does not produce grid lines
    B. Has greater efficiency
    C. Provides better contrast
    D. Provides better cleanup
    E. Absorbs all of the secondary and scattered radiation   4:91

68. An exposure that produces many photoelectric interactions will
    probably result in
    A. Increased fog
    B. Increased scattered radiation
    C. Increased subject contrast
    D. Decreased subject contrast
    E. Excessive penetration of the part   4:80

69. Kilovoltage directly regulates
    A. Definition
    B. Exposure time
    C. Beam wavelength
    D. Tube current
    E. Filament current   4:72

70. As x-ray tube kilovoltage increases, the quality of energy con-
    version _____, the number of photons _____, and part
    penetration _____.
    A. Increases, increases, increases
    B. Decreases, decreases, decreases
    C. Increases, decreases, increases
    D. Decreases, increases, decreases
    E. Increases, increases, decreases   4:64

71. The milliamperage for a specific exposure has a pronounced
    effect on which of the following?
    I.   Part penetration
    II. Radiographic density
    III. Patient exposure
    A. I
    B. I, II
    C. I, II, III
    D. II, III
    E. III   4:49

72. Correct statements about phototiming include
    I.   The primary advantage of phototiming is consistent density
    II. When using the phototimer, it is not necessary to set the
         manual timer
    III. Phototiming equipment improves departmental efficiency
    A. I, II
    B. I, III
    C. II, III
    D. I, II, III
    E. II   4:46

73. Screen unsharpness is affected by which of the following?
    I.   Atmospheric temperature
    II. Relative humidity
    III. Thickness of the active layer
    A. I
    B. I, II
    C. I, II, III
    D. II, III
    E. III   4:38

74. Constituents of the radiographic film emulsion include
    I.   Gelatin
    II. Silver bromide
    III. Lanthanum oxybromide
    A. I
    B. I, II
    C. I, II, III
    D. II, III
    E. III   4:19

75. Which of the following best describes the effect of developer underreplenishment on a radiograph?
     A. Increased contrast, decreased density and increased visibility of detail
     B. Decreased contrast, decreased density, and decreased visibility of detail
     C. Decreased contrast, increased density, and increased visibility of detail
     D. Decreased contrast, increased density, and decreased visibility of detail
     E. Increased contrast, increased density, and increased visibility of detail   4:12

76. The useful density range for medical radiography is
     A. 0.05 to 2.5
     B. 0.15 to 2.0
     C. 0.25 to 2.0
     D. 0.25 to 3.5
     E. 2.5 to 3.0   4:11

77. Radiographic balance refers primarily to the relationship between
     A. Density and contrast
     B. Density and distortion
     C. Definition and distortion
     D. Contrast and definition
     E. Contrast and distortion   4:3

78. Select the set of technical factors that will produce the greatest density

	MA	Time in sec	KV	FFD in inches	Grid Ratio	
A.	600	.15	60	36	12:1	
B.	800	.08	80	55	8:1	
C.	1200	.20	70	72	16:1	
D.	200	.30	80	45	5:1	
E.	200	.06	60	72	12:1	5:311

79. The material most often used for grid interspaces is
     A. Cardboard
     B. Magnesium
     C. Wood fiber
     D. Carbon fiber
     E. Aluminum   5:244

80. In terms of volume per patient, the most consistent major body substance is
     A. Air
     B. Fat
     C. Muscle
     D. Fluid
     E. Bone   5:212

81. The amount of scattered radiation produced during a radiographic exposure is dependent on which of the following?
    I. Tissue density
    II. Tissue thickness
    III. Field size
    A. I
    B. I, II
    C. I, II, III
    D. II, III
    E. III   5:191

82. Radiographic procedures which require that size and shape distortion be kept to an absolute minimum include
    I. Pelvimetry
    II. Radium implant localization
    III. Os calcis
    A. I
    B. I, II
    C. I, II, III
    D. II, III
    E. III   5:170

83. Spiking of the MA meter during an exposure may be due to
    A. Improper seating of the KV selector
    B. Improper seating of the MA selector
    C. An improperly calibrated timing mechanism
    D. Rectifier failure
    E. A gassy x-ray tube   5:119

84. The devices in a film processor which assure that the film will remain properly aligned from one set of rollers to the next are called
    A. Entrance rollers
    B. Microswitches
    C. Turnaround systems
    D. Guide shoes
    E. Worm gears   5:55

85. When the term plus density is used in reference to a radiograph, it usually means that
    A. There was increased absorption of radiation
    B. There was decreased absorption of radiation
    C. There were dust particles in the cassette
    D. There were dirt particles on the front of the cassette
    E. The x-ray tube was improperly centered   15:10

86. An increase in the effective atomic number of an anatomical part would necessitate a (an)
    A. Increase in KVP
    B. Decrease in KVP
    C. Increase is MAS
    D. Decrease in MAS
    E. Increase in FFD   10:33

87. In critiquing a radiograph, it is found that density is approx-
    imately 50 percent greater than desired. If the original
    exposure time was 1/8 second, the new exposure time for correct
    radiographic density is _____ second.
    A. 1/64
    B. 1/32
    C. 1/16
    D. 1/4
    E. 1/2   4:104

88. Correct statements about grid cutoff include
    I.   The most frequent cause of grid cutoff is incorrect
         technical factors
    II. During stereoradiography, grid cutoff is likely to occur
         if the tube is shifted across the lead strips
    III. Grid cutoff is actually decreased radiographic density
         due to absorption of radiation
    A. I, II
    B. I, III
    C. II, III
    D. I, II, III
    E. I   4:85

89. The production of scattered radiation would be greatest in which
    body substance?
    A. Water
    B. Air
    C. Skin
    D. Fat
    E. Bone   4:74

90. Which of the following will increase when kilovoltage is increased?
    I.   Exposure latitude
    II. Patient dose
    III. Part penetration
    A. I
    B. I, II
    C. I, II, III
    D. II, III
    E. III   4:66

91. The effective focal spot may also be called the
    A. Projected focal spot
    B. Actual focal spot
    C. Focal track
    D. Target
    E. Anode   4:61

92. An original FFD is 40 inches and the beam intensity is 1/2 r/hr.
    If the FFD is changed to 60 inches, the new beam intensity will
    be _____ r/hr.
    A. 0.17
    B. 0.22
    C. 0.57
    D. 1.0
    E. 2.0   4:52

93. For a posteroanterior projection of the chest, the mediastinum
     should be over the photo pickup. If the right lung is over the
     photo pickup, the resultant radiograph will demonstrate
     A. Decreased density
     B. Increased density
     C. Decreased motion
     D. Increased motion
     E. No change   4:48

94. If a current of 250 MA is being used, it is the equivalent of
     _____ ampere(s).
     A. 0.0025
     B. 0.025
     C. 0.25
     D. 2.5
     E. 25   4:41

95. Correct statements about darkroom safelights include
      I. The most commonly used safelight filter is the Wratten 6-B
     II. The type of safelight depends on the type of film used in
          the department
    III. Some types of film emulsion do not permit the use of a
          safelight
     A. I, II
     B. I, III
     C. II, III
     D. I, II, III
     E. I   4:24

96. Useful radiographic densities include
      I. 0.1
     II. 1.0
    III. 10
     A. I
     B. II
     C. III
     D. I, II
     E. I, II, III   4:11

97. All of the following are directly influenced by KVP except
     A. Subject contrast
     B. Production of scattered radiation
     C. Radiographic contrast
     D. Radiographic density
     E. Radiographic distortion   4:12

98. The sections of a typical H and D curve include the
      I. Toe
     II. Average gradient
    III. Shoulder
     A. I, II
     B. I, III
     C. II, III
     D. I, II, III
     E. II   4:6

99. Determine the missing factor that will produce the same density
    as the original technical factors.

    | 200 MA | | 400 MA |
    | .70 second | | ___ second |
    | 100 KV | to | 115 KV |
    | 5:1 grid | | Nongrid |
    | 72-inch SID | | 50-inch SID |

    A. .03
    B. .05
    C. .15
    D. .20
    E. .30   5:311

100. Results of decreasing KVP include all of the following <u>except</u>
    A. An increase in total absorption interactions
    B. An increase in subject contrast
    C. An increase in radiographic contrast
    D. A decrease in scattered radiation
    E. An increase in the half-value layer   5:197

101. The projected x-ray beam has a direct influence on which of the
    following?
      I. Object shape
     II. Object size
    III. Object location on the radiograph
    A. I
    B. II
    C. III
    D. I, II
    E. I, II, III   5:134

102. The quantity of remnant radiation is determined by which of the
    following?
      I. KVP
     II. Quantity of primary photons
    III. Amount of absorption of the body

    A. I
    B. I, II
    C. I, II, III
    D. II, III
    E. III   5:15

103. All of the following conditions may be responsible for poor
    screen-film contact <u>except</u>
    A. A cracked cassette frame
    B. Plaster on the cassette front
    C. A warped cassette
    D. Broken cassette latches
    E. The weight of a patient   15:128

104. Nonscreen film is most sensitive to
    A. Blue-violet light
    B. Green light
    C. White light
    D. Direct radiation
    E. Secondary radiation   10:19

105. If a change in part penetration is required, the primary factor
     to change is
     A. Exposure time
     B. MA
     C. KVP
     D. FFD
     E. MAS   10:33

106. The intensity of secondary and scattered radiation is affected by
     I.   Filtration
     II. KVP
     III. Patient factors
     A. I
     B. I, II
     C. I, II, III
     D. II, III
     E. III   4:91

107. Kilovoltage has considerable influence on all of the following
     except
     A. Subject contrast
     B. X-ray beam wavelength
     C. Part penetration
     D. X-ray beam frequency
     E. X-ray beam velocity   4:71

108. Correct statements about the x-ray tube kilovoltage include
     I.   It is determined by the line potential
     II. It provides the electrons in the x-ray tube with kinetic
          energy
     III. It controls the quality of the x-ray beam
     A. I
     B. II
     C. III
     D. I, III
     E. I, II, III   4:64

109. All of the following are major geometric factors in radiography
     except
     A. Object-film distance
     B. Focal-film distance
     C. Angle of central ray
     D. Focal spot size
     E. Grid ratio   4:57

110. A milliamperage setting of 500 is equal to _____ ampere(s)
     A. 0.5
     B. 5.0
     C. 50
     D. 5,000
     E. 50,000   4:49

111. The modulation transfer function is a method of
    A. Determining the amount of quantum mottle on a radiograph
    B. Determining screen speed
    C. Determining film speed
    D. Measuring film latitude
    E. Estimating screen unsharpness   4:38

112. The sulfide particles located in the silver bromide crystals are commonly known as
    A. Halides
    B. Sensitivity specks
    C. Latent image centers
    D. Catalytic areas
    E. Ionizing agents   4:17

113. Which of the following is most directly influenced by MAS?
    A. Subject contrast
    B. Radiographic contrast
    C. Production of scattered radiation
    D. Production of secondary radiation
    E. Radiographic density   4:12

114. The radiation that penetrates the patient and produces the latent image is usually referred to as _____ radiation.
    A. Secondary
    B. Scattered
    C. Leakage
    D. Primary
    E. Remnant   4:10

115. Determine the missing factor that will produce the same density as the original factors.

200 MA		500 MA
1/4 second	to	1/10 second
80 KV		70 KV
5:1 grid		____ grid

    A. Nongrid
    B. 5:1
    C. 6:1
    D. 12:1
    E. 16:1   5:311

116. All of the following will result from lack of beam collimation except
    A. Increased production of secondary and scattered radiation
    B. Increased field size
    C. Increased density
    D. Increased contrast
    E. Increased patient exposure   5:243

117. Subject contrast is decreased in elderly patients due to which of the following?
    I. Dehydration
   II. Poor muscle tone
  III. Increased air in tissues
    A. I
    B. I, II
    C. I, II, III
    D. II, III
    E. III   5:207

118. If a specific exposure is made at 40 KV, all of the following will occur except
    A. Photons of low energy
    B. Variation in penetration of anatomical parts
    C. Radiographs with high subject contrast
    D. Radiographs with high radiographic contrast
    E. Radiographs with excessive density due to secondary radiation fog   5:184

119. Why is the lateral projection of the cervical spine taken at a 72-inch FFD instead of the usual 40-inch FFD?
    A. To decrease object-film distance
    B. To demonstrate the C_7-T_1 interspace
    C. To decrease radiographic unsharpness
    D. To magnify the vertebral bodies
    E. To permit shorter exposure times   5:157

120. The reciprocity law may fail at which of the following exposure times?
    I. 1/240 second
   II. 1 second
  III. 6 seconds
    A. I
    B. II
    C. III
    D. I, II
    E. II, III   5:117

For each word or phrase, select the one heading which is most closely related to it. Each heading may be used once, more than once, or not at all.

	Processing Chemical		Function
121.	Aluminum chloride	A.	Clears away unexposed crystals
122.	Acetic acid	B.	Neutralizes developer activity
123.	Ammonium thiosulfate	C.	Maintains chemical balance
		D.	Hardens emulsion
		E.	Prevents oxidation

5:45

124. All of the following factors govern the degree of structural distinctness of the radiographic image <u>except</u>
    A. Focal spot size
    B. Object-film distance
    C. Source-image distance
    D. Kilovoltage
    E. Motion   15:27

125. In order to properly penetrate the average skull, the suggested kilovoltage is _____ KVP.
    A. 45
    B. 55
    C. 65
    D. 85
    E. 105   10:8

126. Radiographic distortion and magnification can be decreased by
    A. Increasing focal spot size
    B. Decreasing object-film distance
    C. Decreasing focal-film distance
    D. Decreasing KVP
    E. Increasing MAS   10:88

127. In order to maintain radiographic density when substituting an 8:1 ratio grid for a 5:1 ratio grid, the MAS should be increased ____ times.
    A. 2
    B. 3
    C. 4
    D. 5
    E. 6   4:89

128. The type of photon interaction in tissue is determined primarily by the
    A. MAS
    B. FFD
    C. KVP
    D. Grid ratio
    E. Focal spot size   4:75

129. The level of energy conversion in the x-ray tube determines which of the following?
    I. X-ray beam quality
   II. Subject contrast
  III. Penetrability of x-ray photons
    A. I, II
    B. I, II, III
    C. I, III
    D. II, III
    E. I   4:70

130. In general, the size of the penumbra is directly related to
    A. Radiographic density
    B. Radiographic contrast
    C. Visibility of detail
    D. Image sharpness
    E. Subject contrast   4:62

131. A basic problem encountered with the use of a small focal spot is
    A. Decreased definition
    B. Increased penumbra
    C. Increased distortion
    D. Inadequate heat dissipation
    E. Filament burnout   4:54

132. Which of the following MA and time combinations will produce 20 MAS?
    I.   100 MA, 1/5 second
    II. 200 MA, 1/10 second
    III. 400 MA, 1/40 second
    A. I
    B. I, II
    C. I, II, III
    D. II, III
    E. III   4:48

For each word or phrase, select the one heading which is most closely related to it. Each heading may be used once, more than once, or not at all.

	MA x Time in sec		MAS
133.	100 6/15	A.	10
		B.	20
134.	200 3/15	C.	40
		D.	50
135.	300 2/15	E.	60

4:42

136. Solution contamination is most likely to result from carryover of
    A. Developer into fixer
    B. Developer into wash
    C. Fixer into developer
    D. Fixer into wash
    E. Wash into fixer   4:29

137. The shape of the crystals in the radiographic film emulsion is
    A. Round
    B. Oval
    C. Square
    D. Rectangular
    E. Triangular   4:16

138. As base fog increases, radiographic density will _____;
     radiographic contrast will _____; and radiographic distor-
     tion will _____.
     A.   Increase; increase; increase
     B.   Increase; decrease; decrease
     C.   Increase; decrease; Not change
     D.   Increase; Not change; decrease
     E.   Increase; increase; decrease   4:12

139. An ideal radiographic film would have a base fog value not
     exceeding
     A.   0.02
     B.   0.05
     C.   0.2
     D.   0.5
     E.   2.0   4:6

140. The binder in the emulsion of radiographic film is made of
     A.   Silver bromide
     B.   Silver sulfide
     C.   Calcium tungstate
     D.   Polyester
     E.   Collagen   9:25

141. Determine the missing factor that will produce the same density
     as the original factors.
                    300 MA   _____ MA
                    .12 second   to   .10 second
                    80 KV   68 KV
                    55-inch FFD   40-inch FFD
     A.   150
     B.   200
     C.   300
     D.   400
     E.   1000   5:311

142. Devices which may be used to reduce the number of photon inter-
     actions within the patient include
       I.   Cones
      II.   Grids
     III.   Diaphragms
     A.   I
     B.   II
     C.   III
     D.   I, III
     E.   I, II, III   5:235

143. Results of increasing KVP include all of the following <u>except</u>
     A.   An increase in partial absorption interactions
     B.   More uniform penetration of body parts
     C.   A decrease in subject contrast
     D.   A decrease in radiographic contrast
     E.   A decrease in scattered radiation   5:197

144. All of the following terms belong to the group <u>except</u>
    A. Penetrating ability
    B. Beam quality
    C. Beam energy
    D. Frequency
    E. Beam quantity   5:179

145. If the original beam intensity is 20 r/min and the FFD is 30
    inches, the beam intensity at 60 inches would be ____ r/min.
    A. 1.25
    B. 2.5
    C. 5
    D. 20
    E. 40   5:136

146. Visibility of radiographic detail is determined by which of the
    following?
      I. Contrast
     II. Density
    III. Geometry of image formation
    A. I
    B. I, II
    C. I, II, III
    D. II, III
    E. III   5:18

147. Determine the missing factor that will produce the same density
    as the original factors.
              200 MA   500 MA
              .20 second   to   ____ second
              Par speed screens   High speed screens
              8:1 grid   5:1 grid
    A. .02
    B. .05
    C. .08
    D. .10
    E. .40   5:311

148. The most common radiographic artifact is
    A. Tree static
    B. Crown static
    C. Smudge static
    D. The half-moon mark
    E. The double exposure   15:45

For each word or phrase, select the one heading which is most closely
related to it. Each heading may be used once, more than once, or not
at all.

Part	KVP for Sufficient Penetration

149. GI tract with barium   A. 60
                                          B. 70
150. Small extremity   C. 85
                                          D. 95
151. Paranasal sinuses   E. 110

152. Abdomen   10:8

153. A beam restrictor is used chiefly to
    A. Filter out scattered radiation
    B. Limit field size
    C. Increase radiographic contrast
    D. Increase penetration
    E. Focus the x-ray beam   10:52

154. A grid should be used for radiography of which of the following
    part thicknesses?
      I.   4 cm
     II.   8 cm
    III.   12 cm
    A. I
    B. I, II
    C. I, II, III
    D. II, III
    E. III   4:90

For each word or phrase, select the one heading which is most closely
related to it. Each heading may be used once, more than once, or
not at all.

155. Tube housing   A.   Inherent filtration
                                 B.   Added filtration
156. Below tube port   C.   Total filtration
                                 D.   Thoraeus filter
157. At least 2.5 mm   E.   Compensating filter
      Al equivalent   4:28

158. High KVP is usually associated with
        I.   Short scale contrast
       II.   Long scale contrast
      III.   High contrast
       IV.   Low contrast
      A. I, III
      B. II, IV
      C. I, IV
      D. II, III
      E. I   4:71

159. The use of a small focal spot can result in which of the following?
        I.   Production of greater image density
       II.   Production of greater penumbra
      III.   Severe limits on the capacity of the x-ray tube
      A. I
      B. II
      C. III
      D. II, III
      E. I, II, III   4:63

160. If a part to be radiographed is placed midway between the film
      and the focal spot, the part will be magnified ____ percent.
      A. 25
      B. 50
      C. 75
      D. 100
      E. 200   4:57

161. Increasing MAS for a specific exposure will result in
    A. Increased photoelectric interaction
    B. Decreased photoelectric interaction
    C. Increased radiographic contrast
    D. Increased penetration of the part
    E. Increased patient exposure   4:49

162. Select the set of technical factors that will produce the most heat units.
    A. 600 MA, 1/2 second, 110 KVP, three phase, six pulse
    B. 600 MA, 1/2 second, 110 KVP, three phase, twelve pulse
    C. 600 MA, 1/2 second, 110 KVP, single phase
    D. 600 MA, 1/10 second, 90 KVP, single phase
    E. 600 MA, 1/4 second, 120 KVP, three phase, twelve pulse
                                                         4:44

163. If the protective layer of an intensifying screen is worn away, results may include
    I.   Increased artifacts
    II. Decreased light emission
    III. Decreased screen life
    A. I
    B. II
    C. III
    D. II, III
    E. I, II, III   4:37

164. Correct statements about latent image formation include
    I.   The degree of ionization in a given crystal is influenced by the intensity of the remnant photons
    II. The degree of radiographic density is controlled by the concentration of metallic silver crystals present on the film
    III. Latent image formation involves the process of ionization
    A. I
    B. I, II
    C. I, II, III
    D. II, III
    E. III   4:17

165. A high contrast radiographic film is most useful for which examination?
    A. Arteriography
    B. Bronchography
    C. Mammography
    D. Myelography
    E. Venography   4:12

166. Radiographic density is dependent on
    A. Film speed, film contrast, and the quality of radiation
    B. Film speed and the quantity of remnant radiation
    C. Subject contrast, film contrast, and the quantity of remnant radiation
    D. Subject contrast, film contrast, and film speed
    E. Definition, distortion, and contrast   4:10

167. If the clearing time of a specific film is 7 seconds, the fixing time is _____ seconds.
     A. 7
     B. 12
     C. 14
     D. 21
     E. 30   9:32

168. Determine the missing factor that will produce the same density as the original factors.

100 MA		300 MA
.30 second		___ second
High speed screens	to	Par speed screens
8:1 grid		6:1 grid
40-inch FFD		35-inch FFD

     A. .05
     B. .10
     C. .20
     D. .25
     E. .30   5:311

169. Results of increased coning include
     I.   Increased contrast
     II. Increased density
     III. Increased positioning latitude
     A. I
     B. II
     C. III
     D. I, II
     E. I, II, III   5:242

170. All of the following substances are major absorbers of x-radiation except
     A. Fat
     B. Fluid
     C. Air
     D. Muscle
     E. Bone   5:201

171. If a specific exposure is made at 150 KV, all of the following will occur except
     A. Photons of high energy
     B. Uniform penetration of anatomical parts
     C. Radiographs with low subject contrast
     D. Radiographs with low radiographic contrast
     E. Radiographs with excellent definition   5:184

172. The decrease in radiographic definition which is due to the criss-crossing of individual photons in the primary beam is called
     A. Umbra
     B. Penumbra
     C. Quantum mottle
     D. Noise
     E. Interference   5:142

173. The relationship between exposure time and milliamperage to produce a specific amount of radiographic density is described by the
    A. Modulation transfer function
    B. Line spread function
    C. Inverse square law
    D. Intensification factor
    E. Reciprocity law   5:115

For each word or phrase, select the one heading which is most closely related to it. Each heading may be used once, more than once, or not at all.

Processing Chemical

174. Phenidone

175. Sodium carbonate

176. Sodium sulfite

Function
A. Quickly builds gray tones
B. Prevents rapid oxidation
C. Swells and softens emulsion
D. Controls emulsion swelling
E. Helps prevent chemical fog
                                                              5:44

177. Factors that influence the amount of image magnification include
    I.   Motion
    II. Source-image distance
    III. Object-film distance
    A. I
    B. II
    C. III
    D. I, II, III
    E. II, III   15:27

178. Which of the following devices has the greatest effect on maintenance of uniform radiographic density?
    A. Grid
    B. Beam restrictor
    C. Filter
    D. Intensifying screen
    E. Automatic processor   10:57

179. In order to change radiographic contrast, the primary factor to change is
    A. Focal-film distance
    B. KVP
    C. Exposure time
    D. MA
    E. Focal spot size   10:33

180. If a focused grid is used at a longer focal-film distance than the specified range, the effect will be
    A. Increased contrast over the entire radiograph
    B. Decreased contrast over the entire radiograph
    C. Grid cutoff at the center of the radiograph
    D. Grid cutoff at the edges of the radiograph
    E. Increased density over the entire radiograph   4:89

181. Photon interactions that occur in radiography include
    I.   Photoelectric interaction
    II. Compton interaction
    III. Triplet production
    A.   I
    B.   I, II
    C.   I, II, III
    D.   II, III
    E.   II   4:75

182. In order to increase part penetration, the factor that should
    be increased is
    A.   MA
    B.   MAS
    C.   Exposure time
    D.   FFD
    E.   KVP   4:71

183. Radiographic distortion may be described as a variation in
    I.   Object size
    II. Object shape
    III. Object density
    A.   I, II
    B.   I, III
    C.   II, III
    D.   I, II, III
    E.   II   4:62

184. Which of the following would be considered a fractional focal
    spot?
    I.   0.3 mm
    II. 0.7 mm
    III. 0.9 mm
    A.   I
    B.   I, II
    C.   I, II, III
    D.   I, III
    E.   II   4:57

185. Results of high MA, low KVP exposures include
    I.   Decreased patient dose
    II. Increased patient dose
    III. Decreased x-ray tube life
    IV. Increased x-ray tube life
    A.   I, III
    B.   II, IV
    C.   I, IV
    D.   II, III
    E.   II   4:48

186. Select the set of technical factors that will produce the most
    heat units.
    A.   300 MA, 1 second, 110 KVP, single phase
    B.   500 MA, 1/2 second, 90 KVP, single phase
    C.   600 MA, 1/40 second, 90 KVP, single phase
    D.   1000 MA, 1/100 second, 100 KVP, three phase, six pulse
    E.   1000 MA, 1/100 second, 120 KVP, three phase, twelve pulse
                                                           4:44

187. The major advantage of using intensifying screens is
    A. Increased radiographic contrast
    B. Increased definition
    C. Increased resolution
    D. Decreased density
    E. Decreased patient exposure   4:31

188. Which of the following anatomical areas has a high degree of
    subject contrast?
    A. Abdomen
    B. Chest
    C. Shoulder
    D. Pelvis
    E. Skull   4:10

189. If film is stored beyond its expiration date, which of the
    following will probably result?
      I. Increased density
     II. Decreased density
    III. Increased contrast
     IV. Decreased contrast
    A. I
    B. I, III
    C. I, IV
    D. II, III
    E. II, IV   4:16

190. Average film gradient is calculated between the densities of
    A. 0.10 and 2.0
    B. 0.15 and 2.5
    C. 0.25 and 2.0
    D. 0.50 and 2.5
    E. 0.75 and 3.0   4:12

191. The basic and essential items that a radiographic image must
    possess are
    A. Contrast, definition, no distortion
    B. Density, contrast, sharpness
    C. Contrast, no penumbra, no distortion
    D. Density, definition, no distortion
    E. Density, no penumbra, no distortion   4:9

For each word or phrase, select the one heading which is most closely
related to it. Each heading may be used once, more than once, or not
at all.

192. Neutralization   A. Acetic acid
                                        B. Aluminum sulfate
193. Hardening and shrinking of   C. Water
     emulsion   D. Ammonium thiosulfate
                                        E. Sodium sulfite
194. Clearing agent   9:28

195. Determine the missing factor that will produce the same density as the original factors.

1000 MA		_____ MA
.15 second		.20 second
70 KV	to	80 KV
6:1 grid		12:1 grid
50-inch FFD		45-inch FFD

    A. 100
    B. 300
    C. 400
    D. 500
    E. 600   5:311

196. The most common type of beam-limiting device is the
    A. General purpose cone
    B. Cylinder cone
    C. Diaphragm
    D. Filter
    E. Collimator   5:235

197. All of the following conditions would require a change in technical factors from the usual except
    A. Abdominal obstruction
    B. Cardiac enlargement
    C. Atrophy of bone
    D. Lung collapse
    E. Tendonitis   5:200

198. Radiographic contrast is determined by
    A. Focal-film distance
    B. The amount of x-rays produced in the x-ray tube
    C. The different absorbing properties of the anatomical structures being radiographed
    D. The inverse square law
    E. The heat of the x-ray tube filament and the length of time the filament is heated   5:137

199. The support material of the radiographic film is the
    A. Emulsion
    B. Super coat
    C. Film base
    D. Protective layer
    E. Silver halide   5:30

200. At the anode of the x-ray tube, the kinetic energy of electrons may be changed into which of the following?
    I. Heat energy
    II. X-ray energy
    III. Mechanical energy
    A. I
    B. I, II
    C. I, II, III
    D. II, III
    E. III   5:113

Section 2

Radiographic Positioning, Procedures, and Patient Care

201. Maneuvers which are sometimes used during gastrointestinal
     studies include the
     I.   Valsalva maneuver
     II. Muller maneuver
     III. Babinski maneuver
     A.   I
     B.   I, II
     C.   I, II, III
     D.   II, III
     E.   II   2:426

202. When dealing with diabetic patients, the technologist should
     be prepared to recognize symptoms of which of the following?
     I.   Ketoacidosis
     II. Hypoglycemia
     III. Anorexia
     A.   I
     B.   I, II
     C.   I, II, III
     D.   II, III
     E.   III   16:60

203. For intrathecal administration, a drug is injected
     A.   Into the muscular tissue
     B.   Into the subcutaneous layers of the skin
     C.   Between the layers of the skin
     D.   Into an artery
     E.   Into the spinal canal   16:137

204. Anteroposterior and lateral studies are the routine procedure
     for which of the following?
     I.   Hand
     II. Forearm
     III. Thumb
     A.   I
     B.   II
     C.   III
     D.   I, II
     E.   I, II, III   2:100

205. Factors or devices which should be used for radiography of the
     extremities whenever possible include
     I.   Cardboard film holder
     II. Small focal spot
     III. Close collimation
     A.   I
     B.   II
     C.   III
     D.   I, II
     E.   I, II, III   2:82

37

206. The left lateral position for the chest should be utilized
for which of the following conditions?
I. The patient is asymptomatic
II. The patient has severe pains in the left chest
III. The patient has a history of pneumonia in the right lung
A. I
B. I, II
C. I, II, III
D. I, III
E. II   2:39

207. Terms which may be used to refer to the special projections for
visualization of the intercondyloid fossa include
I. Tunnel position
II. Semiaxial
III. Sunrise
A. I
B. I, II
C. I, II, III
D. I, III
E. II   2:166

208. For the lateral position of the paranasal sinuses, the central
ray should be directed to the
A. Nasion
B. Glabella
C. External auditory meatus
D. Outer canthus
E. Acanthion   2:255

209. The terms <u>semiaxial</u> <u>transcranial</u> and <u>lateral</u> <u>transcranial</u> refer
to projections for the
A. Mandible
B. Auditory ossicles
C. Petrous pyramids
D. Mastoid process
E. Temporomandibular joint   2:251

210. Planes or lines which should be perpendicular to the film for a
semiaxial AP projection of the skull include
I. Orbitomeatal
II. Midsagittal
III. Interpupillary
A. I
B. I, II
C. I, II, III
D. II, III
E. III   2:204

211. For radiography of the sternum in the RAO position, which of
     the following techniques will be useful?
     I.   Short FFD
     II. Long exposure time
     III. Deep breathing
     IV. High KVP
     A.   I, II
     B.   I, II, III
     C.   I, II, III, IV
     D.   I, II, IV
     E.   I, III   2:325

212. Routine positions or projections for a cardiac series include
     all of the following <u>except</u> the
     A.   PA
     B.   Left lateral
     C.   Right lateral
     D.   RAO
     E.   LAO   2:428

213. Methods which may be used to enhance filling of the pelvis and
     calyces during urography include
     I.   The Trendelenburg position
     II. Ureteric compression
     III. Rapid shallow breathing
     A.   I
     B.   I, II
     C.   I, II, III
     D.   II, III
     E.   III   2:511

214. During bronchography, the contrast medium is distributed
     throughout the bronchial tree by
     A.   Pressure injection
     B.   Changes in body position
     C.   Hydrostatic pressure
     D.   Osmosis
     E.   Cellular diffusion   2:530

215. The joint most often examined by arthrography is the
     A.   Shoulder
     B.   Hip
     C.   Temporomandibular joint
     D.   Elbow
     E.   Knee   2:536

216. If positioning directions indicate that the central ray should
     exit at a point 3/4 inch anterior and 3/4 inch superior to the
     EAM, the procedure being performed is probably a (an)
     A.   AP skull
     B.   PA skull
     C.   Lateral skull
     D.   Submentrovertical skull
     E.   Half axial skull   11:64

✓ 217. The posteroanterior projection to demonstrate the mandibular
         condyles below the cranial floor requires a central ray
         angulation of
         A.   12° cephalad
         B.   12° caudad
         C.   23° cephalad
         D.   23° caudad
         E.   35° caudad   11:144

218. A grid cassette is most likely to be used for radiography of the
         A.   Hip in the operating room
         B.   Hand through plaster
         C.   Foot through plaster
         D.   Knee
         E.   Elbow   6:142

219. In order to obtain the least magnification for a lateral pro-
         jection of the thumb, which surface of the wrist or hand should
         be closest to the film?
         A.   Radial surface
         B.   Ulnar surface
         C.   Palmar surface
         D.   Dorsal surface
         E.   Plantar surface   2:82

For each word or phrase, select the one heading which is most closely
related to it. Each heading may be used once, more than once, or
not at all.

220. Toward head *D*   A.   Proximal
                                    B.   Distal
221. Toward feet *E*   C.   Medial
                                    D.   Superior
222. Near source *A*   E.   Inferior

223. Away from source *B*   2:22

224. If the patient is in a sitting position with his body and head
         elevated 45°, he is said to be in _____ position.
         A.   An erect
         B.   A seated
         C.   Sims'
         D.   Fowler's
         E.   The lithotomy   16:19

225. A surgical procedure to form an artificial opening through the
         abdominal wall in order to allow for the passage of urine or
         feces is a (an)
         A.   Ostomy
         B.   Otomy
         C.   Ectomy
         D.   Atrophy
         E.   Opathy   16:77

226. All of the following are signs of circulatory impairment <u>except</u>
    A. Coldness
    B. Numbness
    C. Nausea
    D. Pale or bluish skin color
    E. Inability to move fingers or toes   16:170

227. Important points to remember when positioning a forearm for a lateral projection include
    I. The elbow should be hyperflexed
    II. The hand and wrist should be in a true lateral position
    III. The arm should be completely abducted
    A. I
    B. II
    C. III
    D. I, II
    E. I, II, III   2:101

228. The degree of rotation for an oblique hand radiograph is _____ degrees.
    A. 15
    B. 25
    C. 35
    D. 45
    E. 60   2:86

229. Reasons why chest radiographs should be taken in an erect position at a FFD of 72 inches include
    I. To minimize magnification
    II. To show air-fluid levels
    III. To ensure that the great vessels are filled with blood
    A. I
    B. II
    C. III
    D. I, II
    E. I, II, III   2:38

230. Intensifying screens should be used if the body part measures more than _____ cm.
    A. 2
    B. 4
    C. 6
    D. 8
    E. 10   2:99

For each word or phrase, select the one heading which is most closely related to it. Each heading may be used once, more than once, or not at all.

Best demonstrates	Position
231. Sphenoid sinuses	A. Waters
	B. Law
232. Maxillary sinuses	C. Caldwell
	D. Lateral
233. Frontal sinuses	E. Mayer
234. All paranasal sinuses	2:253

235. Parts of the face which should be touching the tabletop for
     the Rhese position include the
     I.   Forehead
     II. Cheek
     III. Nose
     A.   I
     B.   I, II
     C.   I, II, III
     D.   II, III
     E.   III   2:232

236. All of the following positions or projections are typically
     included in a routine skull series <u>except</u> the
     A.   Semiaxial AP
     B.   Submentovertical
     C.   PA
     D.   AP
     E.   Lateral   2:202

Refer to this list for the next 4 questions.
     I.   Lateral
     II. 45° oblique
     III. Anteroposterior
     IV. Posteroanterior
     V.   70° oblique

237. The intervertebral foramina of the lumbar spine would be best
     demonstrated by
     A.   I
     B.   II
     C.   III
     D.   IV
     E.   V   2:302

238. The intervertebral foramina of the thoracic spine would be best
     demonstrated by
     A.   I
     B.   II
     C.   III
     D.   IV
     E.   V   2:302

239. The intervertebral foramina of the cervical spine would be best
     demonstrated by
     A.   I
     B.   II
     C.   III
     D.   IV
     E.   V   2:302

240. Positions or projections which would be included for a routine
     study of the lumbar vertebrae include
     A.   I, II, V
     B.   I, II, III
     C.   I, III, V
     D.   I, IV, V
     E.   I, III   2:281

241. Esophageal reflux may be demonstrated by which of the following maneuvers?
    I. Babinski maneuver
    II. Toe-touch maneuver
    III. Water test
    A. I
    B. I, II
    C. I, II, III
    D. II, III
    E. III   2:426

242. The degree of obliquity for the posterior obliques during excretory urography is usually _____ degrees.
    A. 10
    B. 20
    C. 30
    D. 40
    E. 60   2:518

243. Fluoroscopic control is necessary for which of the following procedures?
    I. Bronchial brush biopsy
    II. Percutaneous lung biopsy
    III. Laryngography
    A. I
    B. I, II
    C. I, II, III
    D. II, III
    E. III   2:530

244. Soft tissue structures of joints that may be demonstrated by arthrography include
    I. Ligaments
    II. Articular cartilage
    III. Bursae
    IV. Menisci
    A. I, II
    B. III, IV
    C. I, II, III
    D. I, II, III, IV
    E. IV   2:536

245. For the Towne position of the skull, the patient is in the _____ position.
    A. Supine
    B. Prone
    C. Laterally recumbent
    D. Oblique
    E. Trendelenburg   11:68

246. Ultrasonography is preferred over radiography to demonstrate which of the following?
     I.   Multiple pregnancy
     II. Fetal death
     III. Fetal age
     A. I
     B. II
     C. III
     D. I, II
     E. I, II, III   6:734

247. Tomography would be used to best advantage to demonstrate
     A. A congenital hip dislocation through plaster
     B. The mitral valve
     C. A subdural hematoma
     D. A Colle's fracture
     E. A March fracture   6:140

248. In order to best demonstrate the glenohumeral interspace, the patient should be in which position?
     A. Prone
     B. Supine
     C. Oblique
     D. Lateral
     E. Erect   2:120

249. Diplococci, streptococci and staphylococci are types of
     A. Yeasts
     B. Molds
     C. Fungi
     D. Viruses
     E. Bacteria   16:14

250. Which type of shock is caused by severe systemic infections?
     A. Cardiogenic
     B. Neurogenic
     C. Hypovolemic
     D. Septic
     E. Anaphylactic   16:59

For each word or phrase, select the one heading which is most closely related to it. Each heading may be used once, more than once, or not at all.

Pertaining to	Term
251. Eye	A. Oral
	B. Otic
252. Ear	C. Buccal
	D. Ophthalmic
253. Cheek	E. Integumentary
	16:126

254. Basic positions or projections of the thumb include the
    I. PA
   II. AP
  III. Lateral
    A. I
    B. II
    C. III
    D. I, III
    E. II, III   2:82

255. Areas which should be superimposed for a lateral chest radiograph include
    I. The left and right hilus shadows
   II. The left and right costophrenic angles
  III. The left and right anterior ribs
    A. I
    B. II
    C. III
    D. II, III
    E. I, II, III   2:39

256. Important positioning landmarks of the pelvis include the
    I. Greater sciatic notch
   II. Ischial spine
  III. Anterior superior iliac spine
    A. I
    B. I, II
    C. I, II, III
    D. II, III
    E. III   2:178

257. A plantodorsal projection is the standard method for radiographing the
    A. Foot
    B. Ankle
    C. Tarsal bones
    D. Subtalar joint
    E. Os calcis   2:144

258. The position or projection which may be used to demonstrate the condyloid processes and upper rami of the mandible is the
    A. Waters
    B. Stenvers
    C. Towne
    D. Caldwell
    E. Rhese   2:248

For each word or phrase, select the one heading which is most closely related to it. Each heading may be used once, more than once, or not at all.

	Divides skull into		Name of plane
259.	Anterior and posterior parts		A. Coronal
			B. Median
260.	Right and left halves		C. Sagittal
			D. Transverse
261.	Superior and inferior parts		E. Oblique 11:50

262. Structures which should be projected within the foramen magnum
     for a well-positioned semi-axial AP projection of the skull
     include
     I.   The posterior arch of C_1
     II. The dorsum sellae
     III. The posterior clinoids
     A. I
     B. I, II
     C. I, II, III
     D. II, III
     E. III   2:204

263. The translateral hip projection may also be called
     A. Anteroposterior
     B. Posteroanterior
     C. Inferosuperior
     D. Tangential
     E. Axial   2:182

264. For the RAO position of the esophagus, the usual degree of
     obliquity is about _____ degrees.
     A. 15
     B. 25
     C. 35
     D. 50
     E. 60   2:431

265. All of the following are mild reactions to contrast media except
     A. Itching
     B. Transitory hot flash
     C. Flushing
     D. Nausea
     E. Laryngeal edema   2:508

266. Injectable contrast media should exhibit all of the following
     properties except
     A. Low toxicity
     B. High acidity
     C. High opacity
     D. Low viscosity
     E. High miscibility   2:529

267. The most common use of conventional tomography is examination
     of the
     A. Larynx
     B. Odontoid process
     C. Orbits
     D. Middle and inner ear structures
     E. Sella turcica   2:536

268. For the posteroanterior projection of the skull, the central
     ray is directed perpendicular to the film to exit at the
     A. Glabella
     B. Nasion
     C. Acanthion
     D. Mental point
     E. Frontal eminence   11:60

269. An occlusal film may be used for radiography of which of the
     following?
     I.   Superoinferior maxilla
     II. Superoinferior nose
     III. Inferosuperior mandible
     A. I
     B. I, II
     C. I, II, III
     D. II, III
     E. II   11:130

270. The guide wire which is driven into the neck of the femur prior
     to the insertion of a Smith-Petersen nail is called a _____
     wire.
     A. Thompson
     B. Seldinger
     C. Coy
     D. Kirschner
     E. Smith-Petersen   6:145

For each word or phrase, select the one heading which is most closely
related to it. Each heading may be used once, more than once, or not
at all.

271. Movement toward body   A. Eversion
                                   B. Lateral
272. Movement away from body   C. Medial
                                   D. Abduction
273. Away from center   E. Adduction

274. Toward center   2:24

275. An informed consent form should be signed by the patient for
     which of the following procedures?
     I.   GI series
     II. Barium swallow
     III. Cerebral angiography
     A. I
     B. II
     C. III
     D. I, II
     E. I, II, III   16:20

276. The method of choice for sterilizing items that cannot withstand
     high temperature is the _____ method.
     A. Ionizing radiation
     B. Gas
     C. Dry heat
     D. Steam under pressure
     E. Chemical   16:101

277. Devices that are used to deliver oxygen by the low-flow method
     include the
     I.   Nasal catheter
     II. Nasal cannula
     III. Hyperbaric chamber
     A. I
     B. II
     C. III
     D. I, II
     E. I, II, III   16:170

278. Which position or projection best demonstrates the head and neck
     of the radius?
     A. AP forearm
     B. AP elbow
     C. Internal oblique elbow
     D. External oblique elbow
     E. Lateral elbow   2:103

279. In relation to the symphysis pubis, the greater trochanter is
     located _____, and the ischial tuberosity is located _____.
     A. 1-1/2 inches superiorly, 1-1/2 inches inferiorly
     B. 1-1/2 inches inferiorly, 1-1/2 inches superiorly
     C. 2-1/2 inches superiorly, 2-1/2 inches inferiorly
     D. 2-1/2 inches inferiorly, 2-1/2 inches superiorly
     E. 2-1/2 inches superiorly, 1-1/2 inches inferiorly   2:53

280. How many ribs should be visualized above the diaphragm for a
     chest radiograph?
     A. 8
     B. 9
     C. 10
     D. 11
     E. 12   2:36

281. Before positioning a patient for the Settegast position of the
     knee, it is necessary to
     A. Place the patient in a laterally recumbent position
     B. Determine the exact location of the intercondylar eminence
     C. Rule out fractures of the patella
     D. Shield the gonads
     E. Hyperextend the leg   2:165

282. A routine study of the paranasal sinuses should include which
   of the following positions or projections?
   I.   Caldwell
   II. Lateral
   III. Towne
   A. I
   B. I, II
   C. I, II, III
   D. II, III
   E. II   2:253

283. When the Towne position is being used to demonstrate the zygomatic
   arches, the central ray should be directed to the
   A. Frontal eminence
   B. Glabella
   C. Nasion
   D. Acanthion
   E. Mental point   2:230

284. The average measurement of the skull between the frontal
   eminence and the external occipital protuberance is ____ cm.
   A. 10
   B. 12
   C. 15
   D. 19
   E. 24   2:200

285. For the lateral projection of the thoracic vertebrae, the central
   ray should be directed to the level of
   A. T_5
   B. T_6
   C. T_7
   D. T_8
   E. T_9 2:305

286. For the RAO position of the average stomach, the centering
   point is at which vertebral level?
   A. T_{12}
   B. L_1
   C. L_2
   D. L_4
   E. L_5 2:439

287. For a cystographic procedure, the central ray should be directed
   to a point
   A. Just inferior to the symphysis pubis
   B. Just superior to the symphysis pubis
   C. Midway between the umbilicus and the symphysis pubis
   D. One cm below the umbilicus
   E. Midway between the anterior superior iliac spines   2:522

288. Branches of the abdominal aorta which may be studied by selective angiography include the
     I. Renal arteries
     II. Celiac artery
     III. Superior mesenteric artery
     IV. Inferior mesenteric artery
     A. I, II
     B. III, IV
     C. I, II, III
     D. I, II, III, IV
     E. II, IV   2:532

289. Advantages of Digital Subtraction Angiography include
     I. Arterial images can be visualized following intravenous injection, thus decreasing the risk factor
     II. Radiation dose is greatly reduced
     III. The equipment is inexpensive
     A. I
     B. I, II
     C. I, II, III
     D. II, III
     E. III   2:537

290. Structures which are demonstrated with a submentovertical projection of the skull include all of the following except the
     A. Carotid canal
     B. Arcuate eminence
     C. Foramen spinosum
     D. Mandibular body
     E. Nasal septum   11:73

291. Soft tissue radiography is most likely to be used to demonstrate a (an)
     A. Dermoid cyst
     B. Osteoma
     C. Glioma
     D. Lipoma
     E. Pheochromocytoma   6:641

292. Subluxation of the acromioclavicular joint is best demonstrated with the patient in the _____ position.
     A. Supine
     B. Prone
     C. Oblique
     D. Erect
     E. Laterally recumbent   6:62

For each word or phrase, select the one heading which is most closely related to it. Each heading may be used once, more than once, or not at all.

Disease		Cause
293. Valley fever	A.	Virus
	B.	Fungi
294. Herpes simplex	C.	Bacteria
	D.	Anaerobe
295. Syphilis	E.	Parasite 16:13

296. A collection of fluid or blood in the sac surrounding the heart, which causes compression and prevents the heart from beating normally, is
    A. Epistaxis
    B. Pectus excavatum
    C. Cardiac tamponade
    D. Edema
    E. Cardiac arrest   16:57

297. A drug that is used to relieve itching is an
    A. Antipyretic
    B. Antipruritic
    C. Analgesic
    D. Antihistamine
    E. Antifungal   16:125

298. When an iodinated material is used as the contrast medium, optimum radiographic contrast is achieved with a KVP of
    A. 30
    B. 40
    C. 50
    D. 70
    E. 120   2:510

299. The most commonly fractured carpal bone is the
    A. Navicular
    B. Lunate
    C. Triangular
    D. Pisiform
    E. Hamate   2:77

300. All of the following structures should be visualized on a correctly penetrated radiograph of the abdomen except the
    A. Lumbar transverse processes
    B. Aorta
    C. Psoas muscles
    D. Kidneys
    E. Lower border of the liver   2:65

301. Correct statements about decubitus radiographs include
    I.   The patient is lying down
    II. The x-ray beam is horizontal
    III. The position is described by the body surface that is most inferior
    A. I
    B. I, II
    C. I, II, III
    D. II, III
    E. III   2:21

302. For the lateral position of the ankle, the central ray should be directed to the
    A. Midtalus
    B. Lateral malleolus
    C. Medial malleolus
    D. Subtalar joint
    E. Posterior malleolus   2:148

303. When the head is in a true lateral position, and it is necessary to project half of the mandible superiorly, the central ray should be angled
    A. 20° cephalad
    B. 35° cephalad
    C. 45° cephalad
    D. 20° caudad
    E. 35° caudad   2:247

304. For the submentovertical projection of the skull, the central ray must be perpendicular to the _____ line.
    A. Infraorbitomeatal
    B. Orbitomeatal
    C. Glabellomeatal
    D. Glabelloalveolar
    E. Interpupillary   2:205

305. When positioning an anteroposterior pelvis, it is necessary to check the height of which structures from the tabletop?
    A. The ascending pubic rami
    B. The descending pubic rami
    C. The anterior superior iliac spines
    D. The ischial spines
    E. The ischial tuberosities   2:179

306. The speed with which barium sulfate passes through the digestive tract is referred to as
    A. Velocity
    B. Mobility
    C. Motility
    D. Frequency
    E. Flow rate   2:422

307. Which procedure might be used in order to visualize the biliary system on a patient who has had a cholecystectomy?
    A. Intravenous cholangiography
    B. Percutaneous transhepatic cholangiography
    C. Endoscopic retrograde cholangiopancreatography
    D. Hypotonic duodenography
    E. Hepatic angiography   2:488

308. Triiodinated benzoic acid compounds commonly used as contrast media include
    I.   Diatrizoates
    II. Iothalamates
    III. Metrizoates
    A. I
    B. I, II
    C. I, II, III
    D. II, III
    E. III   2:529

309. Lower extremity venography is usually performed to rule out
    A. Anastomoses
    B. Arteriovenous malformations
    C. Aneurysms
    D. Thromboembolism
    E. Venous varicosities   2:535

310. Radiographic examination of the collection of veins lining the
    spinal canal is
    A. Azygography
    B. Spinography
    C. Epidural venography
    D. Computed myelography
    E. Discography   2:540

311. Which position is used to demonstrate the optic foramen?
    A. Pirie
    B. Law
    C. Towne
    D. Caldwell
    E. Rhese   11:126

312. Which of the following respiratory tract procedures would require
    the greatest KVP?
    A. Lateral upper trachea
    B. AP lung apices
    C. Lateral bronchogram
    D. PA lung bases
    E. AP trachea   6:374

313. In order to place the petrous pyramid parallel with the film,
    the median plane should be
    A. Parallel with the central ray
    B. Parallel with the film
    C. Perpendicular to the central ray
    D. Perpendicular to the film
    E. At an angle of 45 degrees with the film   2:260

314. If the median plane, orbitomeatal line and central ray are all
    perpendicular to the film, and the interorbital line and coronal
    plane are parallel to the film, the skull is positioned for a
    true _____ projection or position.
    A. PA
    B. Lateral
    C. Basilar
    D. Verticosubmental
    E. Axial   2:203

315. Factors which the technologist should consider before beginning
    to communicate with the patient include all of the following
    except
    A. The physical state of the patient
    B. The patient's age
    C. The patient's ability to pay for treatment
    D. The emotional state of the patient
    E. The patient's socioeconomic status   16:10

316. All of the following areas are particularly susceptible to skin
     breakdown and the formation of decubitus ulcers <u>except</u> the
     A. Sacral area
     B. Knees
     C. Heels
     D. Palms
     E. Scapulae   16:39

317. A patient is exhibiting the following signs and symptoms: anxiety,
     substernal pain, dyspnea, coughing, hemoptysis and tachycardia.
     This patient is most likely to be suffering from
     A. Hypoglycemia
     B. Hyperglycemia
     C. A pulmonary embolus
     D. Parkinson's disease
     E. Bronchogenic carcinoma   16:172

318. A patient from the Emergency Room is brought to the Radiology
     Department with a possible dislocated shoulder. Positions or
     projections which should be taken include
       I. AP
      II. PA
     III. Transthoracic lateral
     A. I
     B. I, II
     C. I, II, III
     D. I, III
     E. II   2:121

319. Bony landmarks that are typically used for positioning a patient
     for an AP abdomen include the
       I. Iliac crest
      II. Symphysis pubis
     III. Greater trochanter
     A. I
     B. II
     C. III
     D. I, II
     E. I, II, III   2:63

320. General rules concerning radiographic positioning include
       I. Three projections are required for all body parts
      II. Two projections as near 90° from each other as possible are
          required.
     III. Three or more projections are required for joint radiography
     A. I, II
     B. I, III
     C. II, III
     D. I
     E. III   2:27

321. All of the following terms refer to special projections or
     positions for the patella <u>except</u>
     A. Holmblad
     B. Settegast
     C. Sunrise
     D. Skyline
     E. Axial   2:165

322. For the lateral transcranial projection of the temporomandibular joint, a double angle of _____ degrees is required.
    A. 5
    B. 10
    C. 15
    D. 20
    E. 25
                                                                2:252

323. The Waters position is also called the _____ projection.
    A. Nuchofrontal
    B. Fronto-occipital
    C. Parietoacanthial
    D. Acanthioparietal
    E. Mentoparietal
                                                                2:253

324. The average measurement of the skull between the two parietal eminences is _____ cm.
    A. 10
    B. 12
    C. 15
    D. 18
    E. 20
                                                                2:200

325. Positions which would demonstrate the cervical intervertebral foramina on the right side include
    I. LAO
    II. LPO
    III. RAO
    IV. RPO
    A. I, III
    B. I, II
    C. II, III
    D. II, IV
    E. I, IV
                                                                2:311

326. If regular barium sulfate is ingested, it will usually reach the rectum in _____ hours.
    A. 4
    B. 6
    C. 8
    D. 12
    E. 24
                                                                2:459

327. Planes which should be perpendicular to the film for a frontal projection during carotid angiography include
    I. Infraorbitomeatal
    II. Median
    III. Acanthiomeatal
    A. I
    B. II
    C. III
    D. I, II
    E. II, III
                                                                2:374

328. The procedure in which plastic polymers are used to selectively
     block certain blood vessels is called
     A. Dilation technique
     B. Occlusive technique
     C. Percutaneous transluminal angioplasty
     D. Therapeutic embolization
     E. Intraluminal fixation   2:533

329. Nuclear magnetic resonance imaging depends on the behavior of
     the atomic nuclei of which element?
     A. Hydrogen
     B. Helium
     C. Oxygen
     D. Nitrogen
     E. Lithium   2:538

330. Positions which may be used to demonstrate the petrous pyramid
     include the
     I. Arcelin
     II. Stenvers
     III. Mayer
     A. I
     B. I, II
     C. I, II, III
     D. II, III
     E. III   11:78

331. Injection of contrast medium into the median antecubital vein
     would probably be the method for
     A. Epidural venography
     B. Superior vena cavography
     C. Jugular venography
     D. Lower extremity venography
     E. Cerebral venography   6:609

332. Examinations which make use of long exposure times include
     I. Ribs
     II. Sternum
     III. Lungs
     A. I
     B. I, II
     C. I, II, III
     D. II, III
     E. III   4:46

333. The most frequent site of nosocomial infection is the
     A. Urinary tract
     B. Upper respiratory tract
     C. Alimentary tract
     D. Skin
     E. Reproductive tract   16:12

334.   When oxygen is being administered therapeutically, it is measured
        in units of
        A. mg
        B. cc
        C. mm Hg
        D. Liters per minute
        E. Milliliters per hour   16:55

335.   The most common size for an adult urethral catheter is number
        _____ French.
        A. 10
        B. 12
        C. 14
        D. 16
        E. 24   16:123

336.   The most common cause of convulsive seizures is
        A. Uremia
        B. Eclampsia
        C. Tetanus
        D. Brain tumor
        E. Epilepsy   16:64

337.   In the lateral projection of the wrist, the carpal bones that
        are usually located most anteriorly are the
        A. Navicular and pisiform
        B. Navicular and hamate
        C. Navicular and lunate
        D. Pisiform and triangular
        E. Pisiform and greater multangular   2:78

338.   Air-fluid levels can be demonstrated with which of the following
        abdominal positions or projections?
        I.   Upright
        II. Lateral decubitus
        III. Anteroposterior supine
        A. I
        B. I, II
        C. I, II, III
        D. II, III
        E. II   2:71

339.   A patient who is having a dorsal decubitus radiograph is in the
        _____ position
        A. Supine
        B. Prone
        C. Laterally recumbent
        D. Erect
        E. Trendelenburg   2:22

340.   All of the following require 45 degrees medial rotation for the
        oblique study except the
        A. Foot
        B. Ankle
        C. First toe
        D. Second toe
        E. Fifth toe   2:139

341. The semiaxial transcranial projection for the temporomandibular joint is sometimes called the _____ position.
     A. Rhese
     B. Law
     C. Mayer
     D. Schuller
     E. Arcelin
     2:251

342. Fractures which involve the orbits include
     I.   Boxer fractures
     II. Tripod fractures
     III. Blow-out fractures
     A. I
     B. I, II
     C. I, II, III
     D. II, III
     E. III
     2:219

343. All of the following are positioning landmarks for the pelvis and hip except the
     A. Symphysis pubis
     B. Ischial tuberosity
     C. Greater trochanters
     D. Acetabulum
     E. Iliac crest
     2:178

344. The chemical symbol for barium sulfate is
     A. BS_2
     B. BaS_2
     C. $BaSO_2$
     D. $BaSO_4$
     E. $BaSU_4$
     2:421

345. How many hours prior to the radiographic examination are oral cholecystopaques usually taken?
     A. 4-6
     B. 6-8
     C. 8-10
     D. 10-12
     E. 24
     2:486

346. Water-soluble organic iodides are used as contrast media for which of the following?
     I.   Excretory urography
     II. Angiography
     III. Intravenous cholangiography
     A. I
     B. II
     C. III
     D. I, II
     E. I, II, III
     2:528

347. The examination which is usually performed to determine patency
      of the oviducts is
      A. Pelvic pneumography
      B. Gynography
      C. Peritoneography
      D. Hysterosalpingography
      E. Sinography   2:534

348. The water-soluble medium used for myelography is
      A. Diatrizoate
      B. Iothalamate
      C. Selenomethionine
      D. Metrizamide
      E. Pantopaque   2:539

349. The position which demonstrates the sphenoid sinuses within the
      region of the open mouth is the
      A. Waters
      B. Pirie
      C. Owen
      D. Mayer
      E. Schuller   11:104

350. All of the following may be demonstrated by a plain abdominal
      radiograph except
      A. A hydatid cyst of the liver
      B. Phleboliths
      C. Uterine fibroids
      D. A pancreatic pseudocyst
      E. A dermoid cyst   6:376

351. A patient is supine and the orbitomeatal line and median plane
      are perpendicular to the film. The central ray is directed 40
      degrees caudad. This projection demonstrates the posterior
      arch of C_1 in the foramen magnum. In order to demonstrate the

      dorsum sellae within the foramen magnum, the
      A. Central ray angulation should be increased to 45 degrees
      B. Central ray angulation should be decreased to 30 degrees
      C. Central ray angulation should be decreased to 20 degrees
      D. Head should be adjusted to make the glabellomeatal line
          perpendicular to the film
      E. Head should be adjusted to make the infraorbitomeatal line
          perpendicular to the film   2:204

352. Which of the following positions would demonstrate the pars
      petrosa with the least distortion?
      A. Waters
      B. Caldwell
      C. Law
      D. Stenvers
      E. Chamberlain-Towne   2:260

353. A disease that can be transmitted from one person to another is
said to be
A. Epidemic
B. Endemic
C. Communicable
D. Inflammatory
E. Aerobic   16:11

354. The instrument used for measuring blood pressure in the arteries
is the
A. Manometer
B. Galvanometer
C. Stethoscope
D. Endoscope
E. Sphygmomanometer   16:43

For each word or phrase, select the one heading which is most closely
related to it. Each heading may be used once, more than once, or
not at all.

355. An antiseptic preparation of   A. PHisoHex
povidone-iodine.   B. Iodophor
                                           C. Zephiran
356. A germicidal detergent   D. Hexachlorophene
                                           E. Betadine
357. An antiseptic preparation of
benzalkonium chloride

358. A disinfectant of combined iodine
and detergent   16:111

359. A patient is placed in the prone position with the median plane
and the orbitomeatal line perpendicular to the film. The central
ray is directed perpendicular to the film. The resultant radio-
graph will demonstrate the petrous pyramids
A. Projected below the orbits
B. Projected above the orbits
C. Projected into the lower third of the orbits
D. Completely filling the orbits
E. Projected below the foramen magnum   2:203

360. The maximum exposure time that should be used for radiography of
the abdomen is _____ second.
A. 1/40
B. 1/20
C. 1/10
D. 1/5
E. 1/2   2:63

361. The midcoronal plane may also be called the _____ plane.
A. Midsagittal
B. Sagittal
C. Transverse
D. Midaxillary
E. Horizontal   2:26

362. An axial projection is usually taken for the
    A. Hip
    B. Knee
    C. Ankle
    D. Wrist
    E. Elbow   2:165

For each word or phrase, select the one heading which is most closely related to it. Each heading may be used once, more than once, or not at all.

        Structure of Elbow   Position that best demonstrates

363. Radial head   A. AP
                                     B. PA
364. Coronoid process   C. Lateral
                                     D. Internal oblique
365. Olecranon process   E. External oblique
                                                        2:103

366. For an axiolateral or oblique mandible, the angle between the midsagittal plane and the central ray should be _____ degrees.
    A. 15
    B. 25
    C. 35
    D. 45
    E. 55   2:247

367. Which position or projection best demonstrates the optic foramen?
    A. Law
    B. Mayer
    C. Stenvers
    D. Waters
    E. Rhese   2:232

368. Which line should be perpendicular to the film for a lateral projection of the skull?
    A. Glabelloalveolar
    B. Acanthiomeatal
    C. Orbitomeatal
    D. Interpupillary
    E. Glabellomeatal   2:202

369. The double-contrast barium enema is essential when the physician suspects
    A. A volvulus
    B. An intussusception
    C. A perforated bowel
    D. Appendicitis
    E. Polyps   2:479

370. In which of the following positions would the aortic arch be most nearly parallel to the film?
     A. LPO, 30 degrees
     B. RPO, 30 degrees
     C. LAO, 45 degrees
     D. RAO, 45 degrees
     E. RAO, 55 degrees   2:375

For each word or phrase, select the one heading which is most closely related to it. Each heading may be used once, more than once, or not at all.

Structure to be radiographed   Direction of central ray

371. AP sacrum   A. 10^{0} caudad
                                        B. 10^{0} cephalad
372. AP coccyx   C. 15^{0} caudad
                                        D. 15^{0} cephalad
373. AP lumbosacral joint   E. 35^{0} cephalad
                                                              2:277

374. Radiographic visualization of an abnormal passage or channel to determine the extent of the tract may be called
       I. Herniography
      II. Fistulography
     III. Sinography
     A. I
     B. II
     C. III
     D. I, II, III
     E. II, III   2:533

375. Radiographic examination of the nucleus pulposus is called
     A. Arthrography
     B. Sinography
     C. Herniography
     D. Discography
     E. Myelography   2:539

376. Which of the following skull positions will best demonstrate the epitympanic recess?
     A. Law
     B. Mayer
     C. Stenvers
     D. Arcelin
     E. Towne   11:91

377. Which teeth require the greatest degree of central ray angulation for intraoral radiography?
     A. Upper incisors
     B. Upper canines
     C. Upper molars
     D. Lower molars
     E. Lower premolars   6:496

378. The optimum KVP range for penetration of iodine-based contrast material is
    A. 50-60
    B. 60-70
    C. 70-80
    D. 80-90
    E. 90-100   5:226

379. For the AP projection of the coccyx, the central ray is directed
    A. 10 degrees cephalad
    B. 20 degrees cephalad
    C. Perpendicular to the film
    D. 10 degrees caudad
    E. 20 degrees caudad   2:277

380. Infections acquired within the environs of the hospital are called _____ infections.
    A. Bacterial
    B. Viral
    C. Fungal
    D. Aerobic
    E. Nosocomial   16:12

381. Which of the following pulse sites must be heard with a stethoscope instead of directly felt?
    A. Temporal
    B. Carotid
    C. Apical
    D. Pedal
    E. Popliteal   16:46

382. Chemical preparation of the skin for a sterile procedure includes
    I.   The use of soaps
    II. The use of disinfectant solutions
    III. The use of a friction scrub
    A. I
    B. II
    C. III
    D. I, II
    E. I, II, III   16:116

383. A sexually transmitted disease is spread by
    A. A vector
    B. Droplet infection
    C. Direct contact
    D. A fomite
    E. Indirect contact   16:168

384. In order to determine correct exposure factors for an AP projection of the shoulder, the part thickness should be measured at the
    A. Anatomical neck of the humerus
    B. Surgical neck of the humerus
    C. Acromion process
    D. Coracoid process
    E. Glenoid fossa   2:116

385. Which abdominal position or projection will best demonstrate
      free abdominal air from a perforated ulcer?
      A. Left lateral decubitus
      B. Right lateral decubitus
      C. Dorsal decubitus
      D. Ventral decubitus
      E. Posteroanterior   2:68

386. Stress movements of the foot and ankle are referred to as
      A. Supination and pronation
      B. Adduction and abduction
      C. Hyperextension and hyperflexion
      D. Medial rotation and lateral rotation
      E. Inversion and eversion .   2:25

387. In relation to the knee joint, the apex of the patella is located
      A. One-half inch inferiorly
      B. One-half inch superiorly
      C. One inch inferiorly
      D. One inch superiorly
      E. In the same transverse plane   2:160

388. Which of the following should be parallel to the film for a
      Stenvers position?
      A. Acanthiomeatal line
      B. Interpupillary line
      C. Petrous pyramid
      D. Mastoid process
      E. Eustachian tube   2:260

389. Which position or projection of the facial bones may be used for
      a severely injured patient who cannot be turned into the prone
      position?
      A. Reverse Waters
      B. Haas
      C. Lysholm
      D. Mayer
      E. Arcelin   2:225

390. All of the following structures are well demonstrated on an AP
      projection of the hip except the
      A. Head of the femur
      B. Neck of the femur
      C. Greater trochanter
      D. Lesser trochanter
      E. Proximal femur   2:183

391. It is necessary to use a contrast medium for radiography of the
      digestive tract because
      A. Organ density in the abdomen is approximately the same
      B. The organs must be completely filled for radiography
      C. Catabolism cannot occur without the contrast medium
      D. Anabolism cannot occur without the contrast medium
      E. Subject contrast in the abdomen is extremely high   2:420

392. For the small bowel series, the amount of the barium mixture usually ingested is _____ ounces.
    A. 8
    B. 12
    C. 16
    D. 20
    E. 24
                                                                    2:459

393. All of the following may be used as negative contrast media except
    A. Air
    B. Oxygen
    C. Carbon dioxide
    D. Nitrous oxide
    E. Thorium dioxide
                                                                    2:527

394. A fiberoptic endoscope may be used to study which of the following structures?
      I. Stomach
     II. Duodenum
    III. Common bile duct
     IV. Pancreatic duct
    A. I, II
    B. III, IV
    C. I, II, III
    D. I, II, III, IV
    E. IV
                                                                    2:533

395. Myelography is a radiographic procedure which may demonstrate which of the following areas?
      I. Spinal cord
     II. Spinal nerves
    III. Ventricles
    A. I
    B. I, II
    C. I, II, III
    D. II, III
    E. II
                                                                    2:539

396. Which basal foramen is usually projected into the maxillary sinus on a Waters position?
    A. Foramen ovale
    B. Rotundum foramen
    C. Foramen lacerum
    D. Foramen spinosum
    E. Jugular foramen
                                                                    11:97

397. The procedure which may be used to determine limb length is
    A. Arthrography
    B. Scanography
    C. Sinography
    D. Ordography
    E. Stereoradiography
                                                                    6:122

398. The usual FFD for chest radiography using the air gap technique is _____ feet.
    A. 6
    B. 8
    C. 10
    D. 12
    E. 14   4:58

399. For a lateral projection of the facial bones, the central ray should be directed to
    A. The outer canthus
    B. The external auditory meatus
    C. A point 3/4 inch anterior and 3/4 inch superior to the external auditory meatus
    D. The zygoma
    E. The gonion   2:223

400. Sterilization is synonymous with
    A. Isolation
    B. Disinfection
    C. Boiling
    D. Medical asepsis
    E. Surgical asepsis   16:110

Section 3

Anatomy, Physiology, and Terminology

For each word or phrase, select the one heading which is most closely related to it. Each heading may be used once, more than once, or not at all.

401. S-shaped portion *D*
402. Between hepatic and splenic flexure *C*
403. Sac-like pouch inferior to *E* ileocecal valve

A. Descending colon
B. Ascending colon
C. Transverse colon
D. Sigmoid
E. Cecum

2:58

404. The major divisions of the stomach are the
A. Greater curvature, lesser curvature and antrum
B. Cardia, body and fundus
C. Cardia, antrum and pylorus
D. Body, fundus and pylorus
E. Antrum, incisura and cardia

2:55

405. The small air sacs in the lungs where the exchange of oxygen and carbon dioxide occurs are called
A. Alveoli
B. Bronchioles
C. Bronchi
D. Lobules
E. Segments

2:33

406. Short bones are located in which of the following areas?
I. Wrists
II. Ankles
III. Vertebral column
A. I
B. I, II
C. I, II, III
D. II, III
E. III

2:8

For each word or phrase, select the one heading which is most closely related to it. Each heading may be used once, more than once, or not at all.

407. Largest tarsal bone *C*
408. Second largest tarsal bone *D*
409. Heel bone *B*

A. Navicular
B. Os calcis
C. Cuboid
D. Astragalus
E. Cuneiform

2:130

410. The greater trochanter is located on which area of the femur?
A. Distal, inferior and medial
B. Distal, anterior and medial
C. Distal, posterior and medial
D. Proximal, anterior and medial
E. Proximal, superior and lateral

2:152

69

411. The most inferior structure of the pelvis is the _____; the most superior structure of the pelvis is the _____.
    A. Ischial spine; anterior superior iliac spine
    B. Ischial spine; iliac crest
    C. Ischial tuberosity; anterior superior iliac spine
    D. Ischial tuberosity; iliac crest
    E. Coccyx; sacral promontory   2:170

412. The anterior nasal spine is located on the _____ bone.
    A. Maxillary
    B. Frontal
    C. Nasal
    D. Vomer
    E. Ethmoid   2:216

413. The organs of hearing and balance are housed in the _____ bone.
    A. Sphenoid
    B. Ethmoid
    C. Temporal
    D. Occipital
    E. Parietal   2:197

414. All of the following topographic landmarks of the skull are located in the midline except the
    A. Acanthion
    B. Nasion
    C. Inion
    D. Vertex
    E. Gonion   2:193

415. Transverse foramina may be found in which vertebral area?
    I. Cervical
    II. Thoracic
    III. Lumbar
    A. I
    B. II
    C. III
    D. I, II
    E. I, II, III   2:291

416. The large mass of bone lateral to the first sacral segment is the
    A. Sacral promontory
    B. Body
    C. Ala
    D. Cornu
    E. Base   2:270

417. Peristaltic activity occurs in all of the following structures except the
    A. Pharynx
    B. Esophagus
    C. Stomach
    D. Duodenum
    E. Ileum   2:416

418. The apron-like structure in the anterior abdomen is the
      A. Greater omentum
      B. Mesentery
      C. Fascia
      D. Linea alba
      E. Vermiform process   2:454

419. The interventricular foramen is also called the
      A. Cerebral aqueduct
      B. Aqueduct of sylvius
      C. Foramen of Monro
      D. Foramen of Luschka
      E. Foramen of Magendie   2:347

420. The external carotid artery supplies blood to all of the
      following areas except the
      A. Oral cavity
      B. Nasal cavities
      C. Eye
      D. Anterior neck
      E. Face   2:363

421. Arterial structures located to the right of the celiac trunk
      include the
        I. Common hepatic artery
       II. Splenic artery
      III. Pancreatic branch
      A. I
      B. II
      C. III
      D. I, II
      E. I, II, III   17:176

422. The smallest facial bone is the
      A. Inferior nasal concha
      B. Vomer
      C. Palatine
      D. Lacrimal
      E. Nasal   11:7

423. The outermost portion of the tooth is the
      A. Lamina dura
      B. Cement
      C. Dentine
      D. Enamel
      E. Dental periosteum   6:487

Refer to the following list for the next 3 questions.
     I.   Navicular
    II.   Lunate
   III.   Triangular
    IV.   Pisiform
     V.   Greater multangular
    VI.   Lesser multangular
   VII.   Capitate
  VIII.   Hamate

424. The carpal bone that contains a hook-like process is the
     A. I
     B. III
     C. V
     D. VII
     E. VIII   2:77

425. The carpal bone that articulates with the thumb is the
     A. I
     B. III
     C. V
     D. VII
     E. VIII   2:77

426. The correct order of carpal bones in the distal row from medial
     to lateral is
     A. I, II, III, IV
     B. V, VI, VII, VIII
     C. IV, III, II, I
     D. VIII, VII, VI, V
     E. III, IV, V, VI   2:77

427. The highly porous bone which usually contains red bone marrow
     is called
     A. Cortical bone
     B. Cancellous bone
     C. Periosteum
     D. Medulla
     E. Endosteum   2:8

428. The tarsal bone which comprises part of the ankle mortise is the
     A. Os calcis
     B. Astragalus
     C. Navicular
     D. Cuboid
     E. Cuneiform   2:132

429. The lesser trochanter is located on which area of the femur?
     A. Proximal, medial and posterior
     B. Proximal, lateral and posterior
     C. Distal, inferior and medial
     D. Distal, anterior and medial
     E. Distal, posterior and medial   2:152

√ 430. The length of the external auditory meatus is approximately
_____ cm.
   A. 1.5
   B. 2.5
   C. 3.5
   D. 4.0
   E. 4.5   2:240

√ 431. The opening of the orbit which is located at the junction of the
maxilla, malar and greater wing of the sphenoid is the
   A. Apex
   B. Optic foramen
   C. Superior orbital fissure
   D. Inferior orbital fissure
   E. Infraorbital foramen   2:219

For each word or phrase, select the one heading which is most closely
related to it. Each heading may be used once, more than once, or
not at all.

	Structure	Skeletal landmark
432.	Thyroid cartilage	A. C_2
433.	Upper margin of trachea	B. C_5
√ 434.	Lower margin of trachea	C. C_6
		D. T_1
		E. T_4

2:31

435. The bump at the back of the head may be referred to as the
   I.   Inion
   II. Gonion
   III. Occipital tuberosity
   A. I
   B. II
   C. III
   D. I, II
   E. I, II, III   2:197

√ 436. Which of the following topographic landmarks of the skull is
most inferior?
   A. Glabella
   B. Acanthion
   C. Mental point
   D. Vertex
   E. Nasion   2:193

437. Demifacets are located on which vertebrae?
   I.   Cervical
   II. Thoracic
   III. Lumbar
   A. I
   B. II
   C. III
   D. I, II
   E. I, II, III   2:289

✓ 438. The interarticular joints of the vertebrae are classed as
_____ joints; the intervertebral joints are classed as
_____.
   A. Amphiarthrodial; diarthrodial
   B. Diarthrodial; amphiarthrodial
   C. Amphiarthrodial; synarthrodial
   D. Synarthrodial; amphiarthrodial
   E. Diarthrodial; synarthrodial   2:269

439. The biological catalysts that accelerate the digestive process
are called
   A. Buffers
   B. Acids
   C. Bases
   D. Electrolytes
   E. Enzymes   2:417

✓ 440. The most distal portion of the colon is the
   A. Sigmoid
   B. Rectum
   C. Anal canal
   D. Anus
   E. Cecum   2:451

441. Parts of the brainstem include the
     I. Midbrain
    II. Medulla oblongata
   III. Pons
   A. I
   B. II
   C. III
   D. I, II
   E. I, II, III   2:345

✓442. The juncture of the right and left brachiocephalic veins is the
   A. Jugular vein
   B. Azygos vein
   C. Circle of Willis
   D. Vein of Galen
   E. Superior vena cava   2:367

443. The most inferior portion of the gallbladder is the
   A. Body
   B. Neck
   C. Tail
   D. Fundus
   E. Vesica   17:192

444. Bones which form part of the floor of the nasal cavity include the
    I.   Palatine bone
    II. Maxilla
    III. Inferior nasal concha
    A. I
    B. I, II
    C. I, II, III
    D. II, III
    E. III   11:17

445. Openings of the stomach include the
    I.   Antrum
    II. Cardiac orifice
    III. Pyloric orifice
    A. I
    B. II
    C. III
    D. II, III
    E. I, II, III   2:55

446. The lower concave area of each lung is called the
    A. Hemidiaphragm
    B. Leaf of the diaphragm
    C. Costophrenic angle
    D. Base
    E. Hilum   2:35

447. Irregular bones are located in all of the following areas
    except the
    A. Cranial base
    B. Face
    C. Vertebral column
    D. Thorax
    E. Pelvis   2:9

448. All of the following are basic tissue types except
    A. Nervous
    B. Muscular
    C. Cellular
    D. Epithelial
    E. Connective   2:2

449. The patella is classified as a (an) _____ bone.
    A. Short
    B. Long
    C. Irregular
    D. Flat
    E. Sesamoid   2:150

450. Which structure is located directly posterior to the acetabulum?
    A. Ischial spine
    B. Obturator foramen
    C. Descending ramus of the pubis
    D. Ascending ramus of the pubis
    E. Pubic tubercle   2:171

451. The air cells of the ethmoid sinuses are located in the
     A. Perpendicular plate
     B. Cribriform plate
     C. Crista galli
     D. Labyrinths
     E. Turbinates   2:238

452. All of the following are parts of the temporal bone except the
     A. Styloid process
     B. Zygomatic process
     C. Mastoid process
     D. Petrous portion
     E. Clivus   2:197

453. The cartilaginous portion of the ear may be called the
     I.   Auricle
     II. Pinna
     III. Ala
     A. I
     B. I, II
     C. I, II, III
     D. II, III
     E. II   2:193

454. Which vertebrae have bifid spinous processes?
     I.   Cervical
     II. Thoracic
     III. Lumbar
     A. I
     B. II
     C. III
     D. I, II
     E. I, II, III   2:291

455. The approximate angle of the L_5-S_1 joint is _____ degrees
     A. 5
     B. 15
     C. 25
     D. 35
     E. 45   2:273

456. The longitudinal folds of the stomach, which are most evident
     when the organ is empty, are called the
     A. Plica circulares
     B. Villi
     C. Haustra
     D. Rugae
     E. Trabeculae   2:415

457. From proximal to distal, the sequence of the divisions of the
     small bowel is
     A. Jejunum, ileum, duodenum
     B. Ileum, duodenum, jejunum
     C. Duodenum, ileum, jejunum
     D. Duodenum, jejunum, ileum
     E. Jejunum, duodenum, ileum   2:449

458. Parts of the hindbrain include the
     I.   Cerebrum
     II. Cerebellum
     III. Pons
     A. I
     B. II
     C. III
     D. I, II, III
     E. II, III   2:345

459. Arteries arising at the bifurcation of the brachiocephalic trunk
     include the
     I.   Right common carotid
     II. Left common carotid
     III. Right subclavian
     IV. Left subclavian
     A. I, III
     B. II, IV
     C. I, II
     D. III, IV
     E. I, II, III, IV   2:363

460. The piriform recess is a structure of the
     A. Neck
     B. Pelvis
     C. Diaphragm
     D. Shoulder
     E. Elbow   17:156

461. The back of the skull is the _____; the forehead is the _____.
     A. Paries; philtrum
     B. Philtrum; paries
     C. Occiput; sinciput
     D. Sinciput; occiput
     E. Base; roof   11:5

462. The structures called canaliculi are associated with the
     A. Antra of Highmore
     B. Lacrimal apparatus
     C. Nasal fossae
     D. Hypopharynx
     E. Trachea   6:521

For each word or phrase, select the one heading which is most closely
related to it. Each heading may be used once, more than once, or
not at all.

463. Anterior depression on distal humerus   A. Olecranon process
                                                B. Olecranon fossa
464. Posterior depression on distal humerus   C. Trochlea
                                                D. Capitellum
465. Articulation for semilunar notch of ulna   E. Coronoid fossa
                                                              2:94

466. The common hepatic duct from the liver and the cystic duct from the gallbladder join to form the
     A. Ampulla of Vater
     B. Duodenal papilla
     C. Biliary duct
     D. Common bile duct
     E. Vesica fellea   2:59

467. The structure that covers the laryngeal opening during the act of swallowing is the
     A. Vocal fold
     B. Cricoid cartilage
     C. Thyroid cartilage
     D. Epiglottis
     E. Uvula   2:31

468. Long bones are located in which of the following areas?
      I. Axial skeleton
     II. Appendicular skeleton
    III. Trunk
     A. I
     B. II
     C. III
     D. II, III
     E. I, II, III   2:7

469. The joint between the calcaneus and the astragalus is usually called the _____ joint.
     A. Tarsometatarsal
     B. Metatarsophalangeal
     C. Calcaneal
     D. Subtalar
     E. Intertarsal   2:132

470. Terms which may be used to refer to the cartilaginous pads at the knee joint include
      I. Menisci
     II. Synovial membranes
    III. Cruciate ligaments
     A. I
     B. II
     C. III
     D. I, II
     E. I, II, III   2:154

471. The small structure located anterior to the ear opening is the
     A. Auricle
     B. Pinna
     C. Hilus
     D. Tympanum
     E. Tragus   2:240

472. The roof of the orbit is formed chiefly by the
      A. Lesser wing of the sphenoid bone
      B. Orbital plate of the frontal bone
      C. Cribriform plate of the ethmoid bone
      D. Greater wing of the sphenoid bone
      E. Squamous portion of the temporal bone   2:218

473. The anterior end of the sagittal suture is called the _____;
      the posterior end of the sagittal suture is called the _____.
      A. Vertex; lambda
      B. Lambda; vertex
      C. Bregma; vertex
      D. Bregma; lambda
      E. Lambda; bregma   2:196

474. The number of bones in the cerebral cranium is _____; the
      number of bones in the facial skeleton is _____; the number
      of bones in the skull is _____.
      A. 8; 14; 22
      B. 14; 8; 22
      C. 14; 14; 28
      D. 6; 20; 26
      E. 20; 6; 26   2:192

For each word or phrase, select the one heading which is most closely
related to it. Each heading may be used once, more than once, or
not at all.

Vertebra   Topographic landmark
475. C₁   A. Xiphoid tip
                                  B. Thyroid cartilage
476. C₃   C. Gonion
                                  D. Mastoid tip
477. T₁₀   E. Inferior margin of ribs

478. L₃   2:296

479. The innermost portion of the intervertebral disk is the
      A. Articular cartilage
      B. Meniscus
      C. Annulus fibrosis
      D. Nucleus pulposus
      E. Peduncle   2:268

480. The most anterior portion of the stomach is the
      A. Fundus
      B. Body
      C. Pyloric antrum
      D. Cardia
      E. Pylorus   2:415

481. Causes of mechanical ileus include
     I.   Adhesions
     II. Strictures
     III. Hernias
     A. I
     B. II
     C. III
     D. I, II
     E. I, II, III   2:458

482. Parts of the central nervous system include the
     I.   Brain
     II. Spinal cord
     III. Cranial nerves
     A. I
     B. II
     C. III
     D. I, II, III
     E. I, II   2:344

483. The hypophyseal fossa is also called the
     A. Cranial floor
     B. Clivus
     C. Crista galli
     D. Sella turcica
     E. Orbital floor   17:4

484. The infundibula of the kidneys are also called the
     A. Pyramids
     B. Calices
     C. Renal papillae
     D. Renal pelves
     E. Medial margins   17:204

485. The chiasmatic groove is a structure of the _____ bone.
     A. Ethmoid
     B. Sphenoid
     C. Temporal
     D. Occipital
     E. Malar   11:30

486. Accessory digestive organs include the
     I.   Spleen
     II. Appendix
     III. Liver
     A. I
     B. II
     C. III
     D. I, III
     E. I, II, III   2:59

487. All of the following organs are located in the mediastinum
     except the
     A. Trachea
     B. Bronchi
     C. Thymus gland
     D. Esophagus
     E. Heart   2:36

488. The process by which bones form in the body is known as
    A. Calcification
    B. Sequestration
    C. Fusion
    D. Arthrogenesis
    E. Ossification   2:10

489. Anatomical systems which assist in maintaining the acid-base
    balance of the body include the
    I. Respiratory system
    II. Urinary system
    III. Reproductive system
    A. I
    B. II
    C. III
    D. I, II
    E. I, II, III   2:4

490. The condition in which the tibial tuberosity breaks away from
    the tibia is
    A. Moller's syndrome
    B. Legg-Calve-Perthe's disease
    C. Osgood-Schlatter's disease
    D. Albers-Schonberg's disease
    E. Myopathy   2:151

491. The wing of the ilium is called the
    A. Crest
    B. Prominence
    C. Promontory
    D. Ala
    E. Pteryx   2:170

492. The frontal sinuses are located directly posterior to the
    A. Frontal eminence
    B. Glabella
    C. Nasion
    D. Supraciliary arches
    E. Nasal spine   2:238

493. The horizontal portion of the ethmoid bone is the
    A. Crista galli
    B. Superior turbinate
    C. Cribriform plate
    D. Ethmoidal labyrinth
    E. Middle turbinate   2:199

494. The shape of the orbit is best described as
    A. Pyramidal
    B. Conical
    C. Cylindrical
    D. Ovoid
    E. Triangular   2:217

495. Alternate names for the body of the sternum include
    I.   Corpus
  II.   Gladiolus
 III.   Ensiform
    A. I
    B. II
    C. III
    D. I, II
    E. I, II, III   2:318

496. The central portion of the lamina that lies between the inferior
    and superior articular processes of the vertebra is called the
    A. Pedicle
    B. Transverse process
    C. Lateral mass
    D. Intervertebral foramen
    E. Pars interarticularis   2:271

497. The esophagus enters the stomach at which vertebral level?
    A. T_8
    B. T_{10}
    C. T_{12}
    D. L_1
    E. L_2 2:413

498. All of the following are parts of the colon <u>except</u> the _____
    portion.
    A. Sigmoid
    B. Ascending
    C. Transverse
    D. Descending
    E. Rectal   2:451

499. The proximal portion of the nephron which surrounds the glomerulus
    is called
    A. Gerota's fascia
    B. Bertin's column
    C. Bowman's capsule
    D. Henle's loop
    E. Da Silva's valve   2:500

500. The common carotid artery bifurcates at which vertebral level?
    A. C_1
    B. C_4
    C. C_7
    D. T_1
    E. T_3 2:363

501. The Angle of Louis is located on the
    A. Sternum
    B. Hyoid bone
    C. Mandible
    D. Scapula
    E. Innominate bone   17:118

502. The term <u>nuchal</u> refers to the
    A. Metacarpophalangeal joints
    B. Anterior elbow
    C. Nape of the neck
    D. Curved rim of the external ear
    E. Eyelids   11:5

503. The sustentaculum tali is located on the
    A. Talus
    B. Tarsal navicular
    C. Tibia
    D. Fibula
    E. Calcaneus   6:97

504. The proximal humerus articulates with the
    A. Semilunar notch
    B. Head of the radius
    C. Acromion process
    D. Lateral extremity of the clavicle
    E. Glenoid fossa   2:112

For each word or phrase, select the one heading which is most closely
related to it. Each heading may be used once, more than once, or not
at all.

505. From urinary bladder to exterior   A. Hilus
                                               B. Adrenal
506. From kidney to urinary bladder   C. Pelvis
                                               D. Ureter
507. Endocrine gland at top of kidney   E. Urethra
                                                               2:60

508. The larynx is suspended from the
    A. Body of the mandible
    B. Mental protuberance
    C. Thyroid cartilage
    D. Hyoid bone
    E. Epiglottis   2:31

509. The axial skeleton includes which of the following?
     I.   Skull
    II.   Sternum
   III.   Ribs
    IV.   Vertebral column
    A. I, II
    B. I, II, III
    C. I, II, III, IV
    D. II, III, IV
    E. II, III   2:6

For each word or phrase, select the one heading which is most closely
related to it. Each heading may be used once, more than once, or
not at all.

Articulation with   Tarsal bone

510. Fourth and fifth metatarsals   A. Calcaneus
                                        B. Talus
511. Second metatarsal   C. Navicular
                                        D. Cuboid
512. Tibia   E. Middle cuneiform
                                                         2:131

513. The main portions of the temporal bone include the
     I.   Styloid portion
     II. Mandibular portion
     III. Mastoid portion
     A. I
     B. I, II
     C. I, II, III
     D. II, III
     E. III   2:239

514. The foramen located at the apex of the orbit is the
     A. Foramen ovale
     B. Infraorbital foramen
     C. Optic foramen
     D. Foramen lacerum
     E. Incisive foramen   2:219

515. The vertical portion of the frontal bone is also called the
     _____ portion.
     A. Orbital
     B. Nasal
     C. Cranial
     D. Squamous
     E. Temporal   2:195

516. The widest diameter of the thorax is at the level of which ribs?
     A. 4th
     B. 6th
     C. 8th
     D. 10th
     E. 12th   2:321

517. The column of bone between the inferior and superior articular
     processes of a cervical vertebra is called the
     A. Joint of Luschka
     B. Articular column
     C. Articular pillar
     D. Interarticular column
     E. Apophyseal joint   2:291

518. The parts of the vertebrae which form the apophyseal joints
      are the
      A. Spinous processes
      B. Vertebral bodies
      C. Articular processes
      D. Transverse processes
      E. Laminae   2:268

519. As compared to a sthenic individual, the stomach of an asthenic
      individual may be
       I. Lower in the abdomen
      II. More vertical in position
     III. Smaller
      A. I
      B. I, II
      C. I, II, III
      D. II, III
      E. II   2:418

For each word or phrase, select the one heading which is most closely
related to it. Each heading may be used once, more than once, or
not at all.

      Inflammation of   Term

520. Vermiform process   A. Pruritis
                                          B. Peritonitis
521. Abdominal lining   C. Colitis
                                          D. Ileitis
                                          E. Appendicitis
                                                                    2:452

522. Which of the following structures is most inferior?
      A. Occipital horn of the lateral ventricle
      B. Foramen of Magendie
      C. Inferior horn of the lateral ventricle
      D. Interventricular foramen
      E. Fourth ventricle   2:347

523. The vertebra prominens is
      A. C_1
      B. C_3
      C. C_5
      D. C_7
      E. T_2 17:48

524. The great saphenous vein is located in the
      A. Chest
      B. Neck
      C. Thigh
      D. Abdomen
      F. Foot   17:212

525. All of the following bones articulate with the vomer <u>except</u> the
  A. Ethmoid
  B. Sphenoid
  C. Maxilla
  D. Nasal
  E. Palatine   11:35

For each word or phrase, select the one heading which is most closely
related to it. Each heading may be used once, more than once, or
not at all.

526. Breast bone   A. Manubrium
                                    B. Sternum
527. Shoulder blade   C. Clavicle
                                    D. Scapula
528. Collar bone   E. Hyoid   2:30

529. Examples of synarthrodial joints include
    I. Intervertebral joints
   II. Skull sutures
  III. Interarticular joints
    A. I
    B. II
    C. III
    D. I, II
    E. I, II, III   2:11

530. The secretions of the endocrine glands are called
  A. Electrolytes
  B. Acids and bases
  C. Suppressants
  D. Depressants
  E. Hormones   2:5

531. The tibial spine is also called the
  A. Tibial tubercle
  B. Tibial tuberosity
  C. Tibial plateau
  D. Intercondyloid eminence
  E. Tibial condyle   2:150

532. Terms which may be used to refer to the hip bone include
    I. Innominate
   II. Os coxa
  III. Femur
    A. I, II
    B. I, III
    C. II, III
    D. I, II, III
    E. I   2:170

For each word or phrase, select the one heading which is most closely
related to it. Each heading may be used once, more than once, or
not at all.

Communication between   Structure

533. Middle ear and nasopharynx   A. Aditus
                                          B. Tympanum
534. Middle ear and mastoid air cells   C. Cochlea
                                          D. Eustachian tube
                                          E. Semicircular canal
                                                              2:241

535. The external landmark that corresponds to the petrous ridge
      is the
      A. External auditory meatus
      B. Top of the ear attachment
      C. Supraorbital groove
      D. Mastoid process
      E. External canthus   2:197

536. Structures which are contained in the costal grooves include
      I.   Arteries
      II.   Veins
      III. Nerves
      A. I
      B. I, II
      C. I, II, III
      D. II, III
      E. III   2:320

537. Spina bifida most often occurs at which vertebral level?
      A. T_{10}
      B. T_{12}
      C. L_2
      D. L_4
      E. L_5
                                                        2:271

For each word or phrase, select the one heading which is most closely
related to it. Each heading may be used once, more than once, or
not at all.

Structure   Bone

538. Lateral malleolus   A. Femur
                                          B. Tibia
539. Medial malleolus   C. Fibula
                                          D. Talus
540. Posterior malleolus   E. Os calcis
                                                        2:132

541. The mouth connects posteriorly with the
     A. Nasal cavity
     B. Oral cavity
     C. Pharynx
     D. Esophagus
     E. Palate   2:412

For each word or phrase, select the one heading which is most closely
related to it. Each heading may be used once, more than once, or
not at all.

                                        Approximate angle of
     Shape of head   petrous pyramids

542. Average   A. 35°
                                        B. 40°
543. Short and broad   C. 45°
                                        D. 50°
544. Long and narrow   E. 54° 2:200

545. The widest portion of the large bowel is the
     A. Ascending portion
     B. Transverse portion
     C. Descending portion
     D. Cecum
     E. Rectum   2:452

546. The renal artery, renal vein, lymphatics and nerves are transmit-
     ted through an area on the medial border of the kidney called the
     A. Pedicle
     B. Pyramid
     C. Papilla
     D. Hilum
     E. Fascia   2:500

547. Sinuses of the dura mater include the
      I. Saphenous sinus
     II. Basilar sinus
    III. Straight sinus
     A. I
     B. II
     C. III
     D. I, III
     E. I, II, III   2:367

548. The superior portion of the talus is referred to as the
     A. Capitulum
     B. Trochlea
     C. Crura
     D. Crus
     E. Head   17:108

549. Which of the following terms may be used to refer to the cranium?
     A. Calvaria
     B. Coxae
     C. Vesica
     D. Crura
     E. Azygos   11:3

Anatomy, Physiology, and Terminology

550. Sesamoid bones are most apt to occur at which metacarpophalangeal joint?
A. First
B. Second
C. Third
D. Fourth
E. Fifth
6:3

551. The portion of the scapula which is located most anteriorly is the
A. Coracoid process
B. Acromion process
C. Glenoid fossa
D. Inferior angle
E. Axillary border
2:114

For each word or phrase, select the one heading which is most closely related to it. Each heading may be used once, more than once, or not at all.

Structure

552. Stomach

553. Appendix

554. Cecum

Location

A. RUQ
B. LUQ
C. RLQ
D. LLQ
E. Midline
2:62

555. Which joint type permits the movements of flexion, extension, abduction and adduction?
A. Hinge
B. Condyloid
C. Pivot
D. Gliding
E. Amphiarthrodial
2:13

556. How many bones are contained in the adult human skeleton?
A. 204
B. 206
C. 220
D. 222
E. 228
2:6

557. The number of phalanges in the great toe is _____; the number of phalanges in the second toe is _____; and the number of phalanges in the fifth toe is _____.
A. 1; 2; 1
B. 1; 1; 2
C. 2; 1; 1
D. 2; 3; 3
E. 2; 3; 2
2:128

558. The concavity between the condyles of the distal femur is
     called the
     A. Intercondylar fossa
     B. Condylar notch
     C. Epicondylar notch
     D. Femoral sulcus
     E. Femoral fissure   2:153

559. The organ of hearing is housed in the _____; the organ of
     equilibrium is housed in the _____.
     A. Middle ear; internal ear
     B. Internal ear; middle ear
     C. Cochlea; semicircular canals
     D. Semicircular canals; cochlea
     E. Middle ear; cochlea   2:243

560. Bones which form part of the base of the orbit include the
       I. Frontal
      II. Maxillary
     III. Zygomatic
       A. I, II
       B. I, III
       C. II, III
       D. I, II, III
       E. I   2:218

561. All of the following bones make up part of the cranial floor
     except the
     A. Sphenoid
     B. Left temporal
     C. Right temporal
     D. Ethmoid
     E. Left parietal   2:197

562. The bands of connective tissue that pass through the breast
     tissue are called
     A. Areolae
     B. Alveoli
     C. Suspensory membranes
     D. Cooper's ligaments
     E. Lactiferous ducts   2:332

563. The vertebral arch is comprised of which of the following
     structures?
       I. Lamina
      II. Pedicle
     III. Body
       A. I
       B. I, II
       C. I, II, III
       D. II, III
       E. II   2:266

For each word or phrase, select the one heading which is most closely
related to it. Each heading may be used once, more than once, or
not at all.

564. Lateral curvature of spine   A. Kyphosis
                                       B. Scoliosis
565. Anteriorly convex curvature   C. Lordosis
                                       D. Spondylolisthesis
566. Anteriorly concave curvature   E. Ankylosis

                                                             2:265

567. Aspects of the digestive process that occur in the mouth include
        I. Peristalsis
       II. Mastication
      III. Deglutition
        A. I
        B. I, II
        C. I, II, III
        D. II, III
        E. II   2:411

568. The largest part of the liver is located in the
        A. Umbilical region
        B. Hypogastric region
        C. Right upper quadrant
        D. Left upper quadrant
        E. Right lower quadrant   2:482

569. All of the following arteries transport blood to the brain
      except the _____ artery.
        A. Left vertebral
        B. Left common carotid
        C. Right external carotid
        D. Right common carotid
        E. Right vertebral   2:363

570. The transverse processes of the lumbar vertebrae are sometimes
      called
        A. Rudimentary ribs
        B. Costal processes
        C. Lateral processes
        D. Vertebral extensions
        E. Pedicles   17:58

571. The fimbriae are extensions of the
        A. Arterioles of the hand
        B. Arterioles of the foot
        C. Heart valves
        D. Uterine tubes
        E. Hyoid bone   17:228

572. The most superior portion of the mandible is the
        A. Alveolar ridge
        B. Condyle
        C. Mandibular notch
        D. Ramus
        E. Body   11:44

573. The supraspinatus and infraspinatus fossae are located on the
    A. Vertebrae
    B. Scapula
    C. Occipital bone
    D. Ilium
    E. Os calcis   2:113

574. The abdomen is divided into _____ quadrants, and _____ regions.
    A. 4, 4
    B. 4, 7
    C. 4, 9
    D. 4, 10
    E. 4, 12   2:62

For each word or phrase, select the one heading which is most closely
related to it. Each heading may be used once, more than once, or
not at all.

     Joint   Type

575. Wrist   A. Hinge
                                              B. Saddle
576. Elbow   C. Gliding
                                              D. Pivot
577. Knee   E. Condyloid
                                                            2:12

578. Structures of the integumentary system include the
      I. Skin
     II. Hair
    III. Nails
     IV. Sweat glands
    A. I, II
    B. I, III
    C. I, II, III
    D. I, II, III, IV
    E. I, III, IV   2:6

579. All of the following are diarthrodial joints except the
    A. Ankle joint
    B. Intertarsal joints
    C. Distal tibiofibular joint
    D. Tarsometatarsal joints
    E. Interphalangeal joints   2:134

580. The pelvic girdle contains which of the following bones?
      I. Innominate bone
     II. Sacrum
    III. Coccyx
    A. I
    B. I, II
    C. I, II, III
    D. II, III
    E. III   2:170

581. Correct statements about the stapes include
        I.   It is shaped like a stirrup
       II.   It is attached to a membrane that separates the middle
             ear and the external ear
      III.   It is attached to a membrane that separates the middle
             ear and the internal ear
        A.   I
        B.   II
        C.   III
        D.   I, II
        E.   I, III   2:242

582. All of the following bones make up part of the skull cap except
      the
        A.   Frontal
        B.   Left parietal
        C.   Right parietal
        D.   Sphenoid
        E.   Occipital   2:195

For each word or phrase, select the one heading which is most closely
related to it. Each heading may be used once, more than once, or
not at all.

            Area   Unilateral number of bones

583. Fingers   A.   5
                                           B.   7
584. Metacarpals   C.   8
                                           D.   12
585. Carpals   E.   14   2:74

586. The large muscle located posterior to the mammary gland is the
        A.   Latissimus dorsi
        B.   Pectoralis major
        C.   Serratus
        D.   Trapezius
        E.   Deltoid   2:332

For each word or phrase, select the one heading which is most closely
related to it. Each heading may be used once, more than once, or
not at all.
                                           Portion of "Scotty dog"
      Structure of lumbar vertebra   on oblique study

587. Pedicle   A.   Neck
                                           B.   Nose
588. Transverse process   C.   Eye
                                           D.   Ear
589. Pars interarticularis   E.   Front leg

590. Inferior articular process   2:273

591. All of the following are accessory digestive organs except the
        A.   Teeth
        B.   Salivary glands
        C.   Liver
        D.   Pancreas
        E.   Appendix   2:410

592. The fundus of the stomach is usually located in the
    A. Epigastric region
    B. Umbilical region
    C. Left upper quadrant
    D. Right upper quadrant
    E. Left lower quadrant   2:414

593. The hormone that is produced when fats or fatty acids stimulate
    the duodenal mucosa is
    A. Cholecystokinin
    B. Heparin
    C. Gastrin
    D. Pepsin
    E. Renin   2:483

594. The vertebral arteries are branches of the _____ arteries.
    A. Internal carotid
    B. Common carotid
    C. Carotid
    D. Innominate
    E. Subclavian   2:363

595. The tuberosities of the distal phalanges of the hands are also
    called
    A. Distal tubercles
    B. Terminal tips
    C. Ungulate processes
    D. Phalangeal processes
    E. Phalangeal crests   17:82

596. The principal artery of the neck is the _____ artery.
    A. Jugular
    B. Vertebral
    C. Carotid
    D. Basilar
    E. Subclavian   11:3

597. All of the following foramina are located in the base of the
    skull <u>except</u> the foramen
    A. Lacerum
    B. Ovale
    C. Spinosum
    D. Magnum
    E. Varolii   11:73

For each word or phrase, select the one heading which is most closely
related to it. Each heading may be used once, more than once, or
not at all.

Structure	Bone
598. Pterygoid process	A. Frontal
	B. Nasal
599. Turbinate	C. Occipital
	D. Sphenoid
600. Orbital plate	E. Ethmoid 2:198

Section 4

Radiologic Physics and Equipment

601. Tungsten is used as the filament material in the x-ray tube for all of the following reasons <u>except</u>
   A. It exhibits thermionic emission well below the melting point
   B. It has a high work function
   C. It is easily shaped into a coil
   D. It has a low vapor pressure
   E. It has a high melting point   1:130

602. Materials which may be used for input phosphors in image intensifiers include
   I.   Cesium iodide
   II. Zinc cadmium sulfide
   III. Barium platinocyanide
   A. I, II
   B. I, III
   C. II, III
   D. I, II, III
   E. II   13:239

603. The number of naturally occurring elements is
   A. 88
   B. 90
   C. 92
   D. 94
   E. 96   3:4

604. The device which prohibits electron flow from the anode to the cathode of the x-ray tube is the
   A. Capacitor
   B. Focusing cup
   C. Transformer
   D. Rectifier
   E. Saturable reactor   7:10

605. Electromagnetic radiation travels at a speed of
   A. 3×10^8 meters/second
   B. 3×10^9 meters/second
   C. 3×10^{10} meters/second
   D. 186,000 meters/second
   E. 186,000 meters/minute   7:1

606. The x-rays produced by electron transition from one energy level to another are called _____ radiation.
   A. General
   B. White
   C. Braking
   D. Bremsstrahlung
   E. Characteristic   7:4

607. The chart which gives the maximum allowable values of kilovoltage, milliamperage and time that the x-ray tube can tolerate in one exposure is the
   A. Anode cooling chart
   B. Heat dissipation chart
   C. Housing cooling chart
   D. Tube rating chart
   E. Cooling system chart   7:6

608. In the United States, electrical current is produced at _____ cycles per second.
     A. 30
     B. 60
     C. 90
     D. 120
     E. 240　　　　　　　　　　　　　　　　　　　　　　　7:10

609. When poorly focused electrons in the x-ray tube strike structures other than the focal spot, the result is _____ radiation.
     A. Secondary
     B. Scattered
     C. Stray
     D. Off-focus
     E. Leakage　　　　　　　　　　　　　　　　　　　　7:13

610. The inverse square law is applicable to all of the following except
     A. Radio waves
     B. X-rays
     C. Gamma rays
     D. Visible light
     E. Positrons　　　　　　　　　　　　　　　　　　　7:65

611. The binding energy of an electron depends on which of the following?
     I. The shell that the electron occupies
     II. The atomic number of the atom
     III. The number of neutrons in the atomic nucleus
     A. I
     B. I, II
     C. I, II, III
     D. II, III
     E. III　　　　　　　　　　　　　　　　　　　　　　1:31

612. The current flowing through a conductor is directly proportional to the potential difference between its ends. This is a statement of
     A. The proportionality of constants
     B. Ohm's law
     C. Einstein's equation
     D. The energy theory
     E. Newton's third law　　　　　　　　　　　　　　1:54

613. When EMF is produced in one conductor by varying the value of the current in another conductor, it is known as
     A. Mutual induction
     B. Self-induction
     C. Field production
     D. Current flow
     E. Faradic current　　　　　　　　　　　　　　　　1:98

614. Examples of common semiconductors include
    I.   Silicon
    II. Selenium
    III. Germanium
    A. I, II
    B. I, III
    C. II, III
    D. I, II, III
    E. I

1:140

615. Attenuation of radiation occurs by which of the following processes?
    I.   Unmodified scatter
    II. Photoelectric absorption
    III. Compton scatter
    IV. Pair production
    A. I, II
    B. I, II, III
    C. I, II, III, IV
    D. II, III, IV
    E. II, III

1:186

616. Which of the following emissions will change the atomic number of the atom from which it is emitted?
    I.   Gamma ray
    II. Alpha particle
    III. Beta particle
    A. I
    B. I, II
    C. I, II, III
    D. II, III
    E. II

1:225

617. Fundamental processes in the production of static electricity include
    I.   Relative motion
    II. Friction
    III. Contact
    A. I
    B. I, II
    C. I, II, III
    D. II, III
    E. III

3:35

618. A transformer is constructed with 1,000 primary turns and 10,000 secondary turns. If the input voltage is 120 volts, the output voltage will be _____ volts.
    A. 8.3
    B. 83.3
    C. 1,200
    D. 12,000
    E. 120,000

3:54

619. The kilovoltmeter measures the voltage at which location?
    A. Autotransformer primary
    B. Incoming line
    C. High tension transformer primary
    D. High tension transformer secondary
    E. X-ray tube　　　　　　　　　　　　　　　　　3:119

620. The modulation transfer function is calculated from the line spread function by a process known as
    A. Boolean algebra
    B. Transfer analysis
    C. Fourier transformation
    D. Quantitative analysis
    E. Equating　　　　　　　　　　　　　　　　　　3:221

621. In the x-ray tube, the flow of electrons from the cathode to the anode is controlled by which of the following?
      I. The rate of emission from the cathode
     II. The amount of heat dissipated at the anode
    III. The voltage applied between the cathode and the anode
    A. I
    B. I, II
    C. I, II, III
    D. I, III
    E. II　　　　　　　　　　　　　　　　　　　　13:53

622. Correct statements about three-phase generation of x-rays as compared to single-phase generation include
      I. Three-phase generation permits operation at a higher power level
     II. Three-phase generation produces increased penetration at a given KVP setting
    III. Three-phase generation produces less heat for a given KVP and MAS setting
    A. I
    B. I, II
    C. I, II, III
    D. II, III
    E. II　　　　　　　　　　　　　　　　　　　　13:96

623. In the International System of Units, the unit of exposure is 1 coulomb per kilogram, which is equivalent to _____ roentgen(s).
    A. 0.1
    B. 1
    C. 294
    D. 2490
    E. 3876　　　　　　　　　　　　　　　　　　　7:11

624. The number of complete wave cycles that will pass any point in one second is
    A. Velocity
    B. Energy
    C. Frequency
    D. Wavelength
    E. Range　　　　　　　　　　　　　　　　　　　7:1

625. The portion of the x-ray tube that is bombarded by high speed electrons is the
    A. Filament
    B. Cathode
    C. Anode
    D. Focusing cup
    E. Tube port   7:4

626. The portion of the x-ray beam which passes out through the tube window is called
    A. The extraneous beam
    B. Secondary radiation
    C. Focal track radiation
    D. The useful beam
    E. Off-focus radiation   7:6

627. The process which eliminates the negative AC voltage cycles in the x-ray circuit is called
    A. Transformation
    B. Transmutation
    C. Suppression
    D. Repression
    E. Rectification   7:10

628. The output of an x-ray machine is dependent on all of the following except the
    A. Accelerating voltage
    B. Tube current
    C. Exposure time
    D. Focal spot size
    E. Filtration   7:13

629. Exposure time may be monitored by which of the following?
     I. An oscilloscope
    II. An exposure time monitor
   III. A spinning top
    A. I
    B. II
    C. III
    D. I, II
    E. I, II, III   7:76

630. The SI unit of electric charge is the
    A. ESU
    B. Coulomb
    C. Farad
    D. Ampere
    E. Watt   1:33

631. Opposition to the flow of electric current is
    A. Electromotive force
    B. Potential difference
    C. Inductance
    D. Resistance
    E. Capacitance   1:59

632. As compared to direct current, advantages of alternating current include
     I.   It is easier and cheaper to produce
     II. The value of the AC voltage can be easily changed with a transformer
     III. X-ray production is more efficient with alternating current
     A. I
     B. I, II
     C. I, II, III
     D. II, III
     E. III   1:101

633. Advantages of solid-state rectifiers over vacuum tube rectifiers include all of the following <u>except</u>
     A. They cannot produce x-rays
     B. They do not require a filament heating circuit
     C. They have a long life
     D. They are inexpensive
     E. They require no additives in order to become conductive
                                                       1:147

634. All of the following are part of the inherent filtration of the x-ray beam <u>except</u> the
     A. Tube target
     B. Tube filament
     C. Glass envelope
     D. Insulating oil
     E. Tube port   1:196

635. Correct statements about the protons and electrons in an atom include
     I.   The charges of the proton and electron are equal in size
     II. The charges of the proton and electron are equal in sign
     III. Neutral atoms contain the same number of protons and electrons
     A. I, II
     B. II, III
     C. I, III
     D. I, II, III
     E. I   3:3

636. The electrical pressure that causes electrons to flow through a conductor is provided by
     A. Amperage
     B. Resistance
     C. Wattage
     D. Voltage
     E. Impedance   3:38

637. The recoil electron is a result of which type of interaction?
     A. Coherent scatter
     B. Unmodified scatter
     C. Photoelectric interaction
     D. Compton scatter
     E. Pair production   3:66

638. The maximum time usually available on a cumulative timer for
     fluoroscopy is _____ minute (s).
     A. 1
     B. 2
     C. 3
     D. 4
     E. 5
                                                              3:121

639. X-rays were discovered in _____, by _____.
     A. 1895, Niels Bohr
     B. 1895, Wilhelm Roentgen
     C. 1895, Albert Einstein
     D. 1910, Thomas Edison
     E. 1910, Enrico Fermi
                                                              13:2

640. The time of one complete cycle of alternating current is the
     _____; the rate at which it changes within a complete cycle
     is the _____.
     A. Alternation; frequency
     B. Frequency; alternation
     C. Period; frequency
     D. Frequency; period
     E. Period; alternation
                                                              13:57

641. Criteria for x-ray production include
     I.   A supply of electrons
     II. A positive charge on the electrons
     III. Slow deceleration of electrons
     A. I
     B. I, II
     C. I, II, III
     D. II, III
     E. III
                                                              5:175

642. All of the following are forms of secondary radiation encountered
     in radiography except
     A. Photoelectrons
     B. Characteristic radiation arising from photoelectric inter-
         action
     C. Bremsstrahlung radiation
     D. Compton photons
     E. Compton electrons
                                                              3:67

643. The x-ray spectrum for a specific exposure is dependent on
     which of the following?
     I.   Beam filtration
     II. Tube voltage
     III. Type of voltage supply
     A. I
     B. I, II
     C. I, II, III
     D. II, III
     E. III
                                                              7:7

644. All of the following are classified as electromagnetic radiation except
    A. Radio waves
    B. Microwaves
    C. Infrared
    D. Heavy ions
    E. Ultraviolet   7:1

645. Bremsstrahlung radiation may also be called
      I.   Characteristic radiation
     II.   White radiation
    III.   General radiation
    A. I
    B. II
    C. III
    D. I, II, III
    E. II, III   7:3

646. Methods which may be used to aid in the process of heat dissipation in the x-ray tube include
      I.   Spreading the electron bombardment over a larger area
     II.   Using a larger exposure time to decrease the rate of heat production
    III.   Angling the face of the anode to increase the size of the actual focal spot
    A. I
    B. I, II
    C. I, II, III
    D. II, III
    E. III   7:6

647. When filtration is interposed in the x-ray beam
    A. Quantity and quality of radiation are increased
    B. Quantity and quality of radiation are decreased
    C. Quantity of radiation is increased, and quality is decreased
    D. Quantity of radiation is decreased, and quality is increased
    E. Quantity of radiation is unchanged, and quality is decreased
                                                            7:9

648. Which statement about the photon energy, wavelength and frequency of an x-ray beam is correct?
    A. Photon energy = wavelength x frequency
    B. Photon energy = Planck's constant x the speed of light
    C. Photon energy = Velocity x electron volts
    D. Photon energy = Planck's constant x frequency
    E. Photon energy = wavelength x the speed of light   7:12

649. Secondary radiation consists of which of the following?
      I.   Characteristic x-ray photons
     II.   Photoelectrons
    III.   Compton electrons
    A. I
    B. I, II
    C. I, II, III
    D. II, III
    E. III   7:23

650. The elements whose atoms require one electron to completely fill the outer shell are called
    A. Inert elements
    B. Noble gasses
    C. Rare earths
    D. Halogens
    E. Dielectrics
    1:30

651. A device that is used to measure the flow of electric current is a (an)
    A. Iometer
    B. Capacitor
    C. Condenser
    D. Rheostat
    E. Ammeter
    1:52

652. When electromotive force is being generated by electromagnetism, the magnitude of the induced EMF depends on all of the following except the
    A. Speed of movement
    B. Strength of the wire
    C. Strength of the magnet
    D. Number of turns on the coil
    E. Distance of the magnet from the coil
    1:95

653. Functions of the x-ray tube housing include
    I.   Radiation protection
    II. Electrical protection
    III. Thermal protection
    A. I
    B. I, II
    C. I, II, III
    D. II, III
    E. III
    1:135

654. X-ray beams are _____; gamma ray beams are _____.
    A. Heterogeneous; heterogeneous
    B. Heterogeneous; homogeneous
    C. Homogeneous; homogeneous
    D. Homogeneous; heterogeneous
    E. Polyenergetic; polyenergetic
    1:183

655. When an atom emits an alpha particle, the atomic number is decreased by _____, the neutron number is decreased by _____, and the mass number is decreased by _____.
    A. 1, 1, 2
    B. 1, 2, 1
    C. 2, 1, 1
    D. 2, 2, 4
    E. 2, 4, 2
    1:224

656. If the wavelength of an electromagnetic wave is less than 10^{-6} Angstroms, the wave is probably classified as
    A. Cosmic radiation
    B. Ultraviolet radiation
    C. Visible light
    D. Infrared radiation
    E. Radar waves   3:27

657. Methods which may be used to increase the strength of the magnetic field of a solenoid include
    I. Increasing the current
    II. Increasing the number of loops
    III. Inserting a soft iron core
    A. I, II
    B. I, III
    C. II, III
    D. I, II, III
    E. I   3:52

658. Which type of timer used in x-ray circuits provides exposure time in increments of milliseconds?
    A. Mechanical
    B. Electronic
    C. Synchronous
    D. Impulse
    E. Ionometric   3:116

659. Adjacent structures within a patient transmit 1,000 photons/mm^2 through structure B and 1,350 photons/mm^2 through structure A. The percent of subject contrast is _____ percent.
    A. 0.26
    B. 2.6
    C. 7.4
    D. 26
    E. 74   3:215

660. Quantum mottle may be caused by
    A. High photon fluence
    B. Low photon fluence
    C. Slow speed intensifying screens
    D. Half-wave rectification
    E. A gassy x-ray tube   13:35

661. Examples of nucleons include the
    I. Electron
    II. Proton
    III. Neutron
    A. I
    B. I, II
    C. I, II, III
    D. II, III
    E. III   3:14

662. The target of the electron cloud in the x-ray tube is the
    A. Focusing cup
    B. Filament
    C. Cathode
    D. Focal spot
    E. Tube port   5:115

663. Areas in the x-ray tube which have critical heat capacities
    include the
      I. Tube housing
     II. Anode body
    III. Focal spot
    A. I, II
    B. I, III
    C. II, III
    D. I, II, III
    E. III   13:89

664. Basic controls of an x-ray machine include the
      I. Kilovoltage control
     II. Current control
    III. Spectral control
     IV. Timer
    A. I, II
    B. III, IV
    C. I, II, III
    D. I, II, III, IV
    E. I, II, IV   7:5

665. The SI unit of absorbed dose is the gray, which is defined as
    A. One joule per kilogram
    B. One hundred joules per kilogram
    C. One erg per gram
    D. One hundred ergs per gram
    E. Ten rads   7:12

666. Which of the following statements best explains the relation-
    ship of photon energy, wavelength and frequency?
    A. Short wavelength and low frequency produce high photon
       energy
    B. Short wavelength and high frequency produce high photon
       energy
    C. Short wavelength and high frequency produce low photon
       energy
    D. Long wavelength and high frequency produce high photon
       energy
    E. Long wavelength and high frequency produce low photon
       energy   7:2

667. The liberation of electrons from the negative terminal of the
    x-ray tube is referred to as
    A. Spectral emission
    B. Thermionic emission
    C. Characteristic radiation
    D. Bremsstrahlung radiation
    E. Electron acceleration   7:4

668. All of the following are contained within the x-ray tube housing
      except
      A. Electrical coils for rotating the anode.
      B. Oil for transmitting heat from the tube to the housing.
      C. The evacuated glass envelope.
      D. Lead for shielding purposes.
      E. The saturable reactor.   7:6

669. In a full-wave rectified circuit, the negative portion of the
      cycle is
      A. Inverted
      B. Suppressed
      C. Eliminated
      D. Blocked
      E. Transferred   7:10

670. The kilovoltage range for radiography is _____ KVP.
      A. 10-150
      B. 20-170
      C. 30-120
      D. 50-150
      E. 60-150   7:15

671. When x-ray equipment is checked for accuracy, the actual KVP
      should be within a range of $\pm$_____ KVP of the indicated KVP.
      A. 1
      B. 3
      C. 4
      D. 10
      E. 15   7:76

672. The SI unit of potential difference is the
      A. Newton
      B. Joule
      C. Coulomb
      D. Volt
      E. Watt   1:36

673. Correct statements about the resistance in an electrical circuit
      include
      I.   The total value of resistances in parallel is always less
            than the value of any individual resistance
      II.   When current approaches resistances in parallel, it divides
            in inverse proportion to the value of the resistances.
      III. In a parallel circuit, the potential difference across all
            of the resistances is the same
      A. I
      B. II
      C. III
      D. I, II
      E. I, II, III   1:62

674. Alternating current may be generated by which of the following methods?
    I. The conductor moves and the magnet is stationary
    II. The magnet moves and the conductor is stationary
    III. The conductor and the magnet are stationary, but the strength of the magnetic field varies
    A. I
    B. II
    C. III
    D. I, II
    E. I, II, III   1:101

675. The SI unit of frequency is the
    A. Cycle
    B. Hertz
    C. Farad
    D. Coulomb
    E. Nanometer   1:156

676. Pair production occurs when photon energies exceed ____ MeV.
    A. 0.51
    B. 0.69
    C. 0.76
    D. 1.02
    E. 1.69   1:197

677. Electrons revolve around the atomic nucleus in certain allowed orbits, and no energy is emitted or absorbed by the atom as long as the electrons remain in their original orbit. This is a statement of
    A. Newton's first law
    B. Newton's second law
    C. Einstein's theory of relativity
    D. Bohr's first postulate
    E. The law of conservation of energy   3:6

678. Correct statements about the resistance in a conductive wire include
    I. The resistance will increase if the length of the wire is increased
    II. The resistance will increase if the diameter of the wire is increased
    III. The resistance will increase if the temperature is increased
    A. I, II
    B. I, III
    C. II, III
    D. I, II, III
    E. I   3:39

679. Properties of tungsten that make it particularly suitable as an x-ray tube target include
    I. High atomic number
    II. High melting point
    III. High thermal conductivity
    IV. High vapor pressure
    A. I, II
    B. I, II, III
    C. I, II, III, IV
    D. I, III, IV
    E. I, IV   3:97

680. Silver-activated cadmium-zinc sulfide is a substance which may
      be used as a component of
      A. Intensifying screens
      B. Fluorescent screens
      C. Thermoluminescent dosimeters
      D. Scintillation counters
      E. Radiographic film   3:128

681. All of the following are properties of x-rays <u>except</u>
      A. They can penetrate matter
      B. They can disrupt a magnetic field
      C. They can cause fluorescence
      D. They can expose film
      E. They can cause biological changes   13:4

682. When the focal spot in an x-ray tube undergoes a change in size
      with changes in MA and KVP, the effect is known as
      A. Saturation
      B. Field emission
      C. Electron divergence
      D. Blur
      E. Blooming   13:223

683. A high frequency x-ray photon will exhibit which of the following
      properties?
       I. Long wavelength
      II. Short wavelength
     III. High energy
      IV. Low energy
      A. I, III
      B. II, IV
      C. I, IV
      D. II, III
      E. II   4:65

684. The mass of an object is the product of its
      A. Energy and weight
      B. Size and weight
      C. Length, width and depth
      D. Volume and density
      E. Density and specific gravity   13:27

For each word or phrase, select the one heading which is most closely
related to it. Each heading may be used once, more than once, or
not at all.

685. Determines photon energy   A. Timer
                                            B. Tube current
686. Determines number of photons   C. Resistance
                                            D. Tube voltage
687. Determines period of x-ray production E. Focusing cup   7:5

688. Terrestrial sources of radiation include
    I.   Uranium
   II.   Thorium
  III.   Radium
    A. I
    B. II
    C. III
    D. I, II
    E. I, II, III   7:1

689. All of the following are correct statements about the process
    of x-ray production except
    A. The efficiency of x-ray production is very low
    B. X-rays are produced as a by-product of the absorption of
        high speed electrons
    C. The x-rays produced are monoenergetic in nature
    D. A great deal of the electron energy is converted to heat
        in the x-ray tube target
    E. Most of the electrons involved in x-ray production undergo
        multiple interactions   7:3

690. In relation to the cathode, the face of the x-ray tube target
    is oriented at an angle of approximately _____ degrees.
    A. 0
    B. 5
    C. 8
    D. 20
    E. 30   7:5

691. Factors which affect the energy spectrum of the x-ray beam
    include
    I.   Filtration
   II.   Tube voltage
  III.   Type of voltage supply
   IV.   Milliamperage
    A. I, II
    B. I, II, III
    C. I, III
    D. I, III, IV
    E. I, II, III, IV   7:7

692. Correct statements about the HVL for a specific x-ray beam
    include
    I.   The HVL is a constant quantity
   II.   The second HVL will be greater than the first HVL
  III.   The difference between successive HVLs gets larger and
         larger
    A. I
    B. II
    C. III
    D. II, III
    E. I, III   7:11

693. At the beam energies involved in radiography, scattered photons
      are radiated chiefly in which direction?
      A. At 90° to the scattering object
      B. Chiefly in a forward direction
      C. Chiefly in a backward direction
      D. They radiate equally in all directions
      E. Scattered photons move only in a direction counter to the
          law of conservation of momentum   7:19

694. If the atomic number of an element is 8, the maximum number
      of electrons that can occupy the L shell is
      A. 2
      B. 4
      C. 6
      D. 7
      E. 8   1:29

695. The device which consists of two electrodes separated by an
      insulator is a (an)
      A. Rheostat
      B. Choke coil
      C. Saturable reactor
      D. Solenoid
      E. Capacitor   1:50

696. The strength of a magnetic field in a solenoid may be increased
      by
       I. Increasing the number of turns on the coil
      II. Inserting a soft iron core into the coil
     III. Increasing the current through the solenoid
      A. I, II
      B. I, III
      C. II, III
      D. I, II, III
      E. III   1:82

697. The condition in which all available electrons are being drawn
      across the x-ray tube is referred to as
      A. Thermionic emission
      B. Space charge
      C. The space charge limited condition
      D. Saturation
      E. Rectification   1:127

698. Factors which will increase the intensity of an x-ray beam
      include
       I.   Increased tube voltage
      II.   Increased tube current
     III.   Increased tube filtration
      IV.   Increased atomic number of target
      A. I, II
      B. I, II, III
      C. I, II, III, IV
      D. I, II, IV
      E. I, III   1:180

699. All of the following are naturally occurring unstable isotopes
except
    A. Cobalt 60
    B. Carbon 14
    C. Potassium 40
    D. Radium 226
    E. Uranium 238   1:223

700. Electromagnetic waves possess which of the following?
    I.   Energy
    II. Mass
    III. Charge
    A. I
    B. I, II
    C. I, II, III
    D. II, III
    E. III   3:24

701. Substances which exhibit the property of ferromagnetism include
    I.   Iron
    II. Cobalt
    III. Nickel
    A. I
    B. I, II
    C. I, II, III
    D. II, III
    E. III   3:49

702. In most modern x-ray generators, exposure time is controlled
with a (an) _____ timer.
    A. Electronic
    B. Snychronous
    C. Impulse
    D. Mechanical
    E. Automatic   3:115

703. Image quality is most often degraded by
    A. Excessive kilovoltage
    B. Excessive milliamperage
    C. Excessive exposure time
    D. Patient motion
    E. Inadequate focal-film distance   3:197

704. All of the following are physical characteristics of electromagnetic photons except
    A. Mass
    B. Energy
    C. Frequency
    D. Wavelength
    E. Velocity   13:19

705. Transformer losses that are due to the heating effect of the
current are called
    A. Faradic losses
    B. Capacitance losses
    C. Copper losses
    D. Eddy currents
    E. Hysteresis   1:111

706. The kilovoltage needed to produce an x-ray beam with a minimum
     wavelength of 0.155 angstrom is
     A. 60
     B. 80
     C. 100
     D. 120
     E. 155   5:179

707. The rate of electron emission from the x-ray tube filament is
     dependent on the
     A. Exposure time
     B. Focal spot size
     C. Kilovoltage
     D. Filament temperature
     E. Anode characteristics   13:83

708. Forty inches is the approximate equivalent of
       I. One meter
      II. One hundred centimeters
     III. One kilometer
     A. I, II
     B. II, III
     C. I
     D. II
     E. III   6:902

709. All of the following statements about the photoelectric effect
     are correct except
     A. The interaction occurs between an x-ray photon and a
        loosely bound orbital electron
     B. The total energy of the photon is absorbed
     C. The total energy of the photon is transferred to the electron
     D. The photon ceases to exist
     E. The interaction is accompanied by a characteristic x-ray
                                                                    7:15

710. The thickness of material that radiation can penetrate depends on
       I. The composition of the material
      II. The energy of the radiation
     III. The ionizing effect of the radiation
     A. I
     B. II
     C. III
     D. I, II
     E. I, II, III   7:2

711. The energy range of Bremsstrahlung photons is
     A. Very low
     B. Very high
     C. One level only
     D. From zero to the maximum electron energy
     E. Indeterminate   7:5

712. In cases where low energy photons are necessary for producing
      a radiograph, the x-ray tube window is made of
      A. Glass
      B. Beryllium
      C. Lead shutters
      D. Lithium
      E. Carbon   7:6

713. If the kilovoltage setting is the same, which type of x-ray
      unit will produce an x-ray beam with the highest average energy?
      A. Self-rectified
      B. Half-wave rectified
      C. Full-wave rectified
      D. Three-phase generator
      E. Constant potential   7:16

714. Methods of accurately determining KVP include
        I. An Ardran and Crooks cassette
       II. A high voltage divider network
      III. A spinning top
      A. I
      B. I, II
      C. I, II, III
      D. II, III
      E. III   7:77

715. Materials through which electric charges are not able to move
      are called
      A. Capacitors
      B. Transducers
      C. Solenoids
      D. Rheostats
      E. Insulators   1:40

716. The ability of an electrical supply device to maintain a potential
      difference is
      A. Wattage
      B. Voltage
      C. Electromotive force
      D. Power
      E. Capacitance   1:66

717. The peak value of a 240-volt line voltage is ____ volts peak.
      A. 120
      B. 169
      C. 220
      D. 260
      E. 336   1:105

718. The longest wavelength in the electromagnetic spectrum is
      A. Radio waves
      B. Radar waves
      C. Microwaves
      D. Infrared rays
      E. Red light   1:157

719. The main attenuation process in radiography is _____; the
     main attenuation process in radiotherapy is _____.
     A. Compton scattering; pair production
     B. Pair production; Compton scattering
     C. Photoelectric absorption; pair production
     D. Pair production; photoelectric absorption
     E. Photoelectric absorption; Compton scattering   1:197

720. In the Periodic Table of Elements, each row in the table is
     called a _____, and each column is called a _____.
     A. Family, group
     B. Group, family
     C. Period, group
     D. Group, period
     E. Family, period   3:11

721. If a voltage of 10 volts is applied across a tungsten filament
     with a resistance of 1.25 ohms, the current flowing through the
     filament will be _____ amperes.
     A. 4.5
     B. 6.0
     C. 8.0
     D. 12.5
     E. 125   3:41

722. Stationary anode x-ray tubes are used in x-ray units designed
     for
       I. Dental radiography
      II. Radiation therapy
     III. Vascular imaging
     A. I
     B. I, II
     C. I, II, III
     D. II, III
     E. III   3:98

723. All of the following are components of an image intensifier
     except the
     A. Input phosphor
     B. Output phosphor
     C. Evacuated glass envelope
     D. Focusing electrodes
     E. Thyratron   3:131

724. The most common unit of power is the
     A. Electron volt
     B. Volt
     C. Joule
     D. Watt
     E. Erg   13:13

725. Film dimensions typically used in intensified radiography include
     all of the following except
     A. 16 mm
     B. 35 mm
     C. 70 mm
     D. 90 mm
     E. 170 mm   13:243

726. In the process of x-ray production, the amount of electron
     kinetic energy converted into x-radiation is _____ percent; the
     amount converted into heat is _____ percent.
     A. 98; 2
     B. 2; 98
     C. 99.8; 0.2
     D. 0.2; 99.8
     E. 100; 0   5:177

For each word or phrase, select the one heading which is most closely
related to it. Each heading may be used once, more than once, or not
at all.
         Material   Application in radiography

727. Silver   A. Tube window
                               B. Absorber in film
728. Iodine   C. Contrast medium
                               D. X-ray source
729. Lead   E. Shielding

730. Beryllium   13:32

731. Electromagnetic radiations that are highly penetrating include
     the
       I. High energy radiations
      II. Medium energy radiations
     III. Low energy radiations
     A. I
     B. II
     C. III
     D. I, III
     E. I, II, III   7:2

732. Types of radiation which are transmitted without the presence
     of a particle with mass include
       I. Radio
      II. Visible light
     III. X-rays
     A. I
     B. I, II
     C. I, II, III
     D. II, III
     E. III   7:1

733. An electromagnetic wave with a wavelength of 10^{15} nanometers
     and a frequency of 60 hertz will exhibit which of the following
     properties?
     A. It will be particulate radiation
     B. It will be high energy radiation
     C. It will be low energy radiation
     D. It will be poorly penetrating
     E. It will probably take the form of an x-ray   7:2

734. The most suitable material for an x-ray tube target is
     A. Copper
     B. Tungsten
     C. Lead
     D. Silver
     E. Titanium   7:5

735. In a chart of the x-ray spectrum, the spikes which are imposed
     on top of the spectrum are due to _____ radiation.
     A. Secondary
     B. Scattered
     C. Stray
     D. Bremsstrahlung
     E. Characteristic   7:7

736. The material ordinarily used for HVL determinations in radiography
     is
     A. Aluminum
     B. Beryllium
     C. Copper
     D. Tin
     E. Lead   7:11

737. The energy level at which photoelectric and Compton interaction
     are essentially equal is _____ KeV.
     A. 26
     B. 43
     C. 57
     D. 69
     E. 74   7:19

738. All of the following are classified as elements except
     A. Hydrogen
     B. Carbon
     C. Oxygen
     D. Urea
     E. Nitrogen   1:23

739. The unit of capacitance is the
     A. Volt
     B. Coulomb
     C. Ampere
     D. Ohm
     E. Farad   1:44

740. Correct statements about magnetic lines of force include
    I.   A line of force originates at the north pole and ends at the south pole
    II. No two lines of force ever cross each other
    III. The lines of force are most concentrated near the poles
    A.   I
    B.   I, II
    C.   I, II, III
    D.   II, III
    E.   III   1:77

741. A device which acts as a conductor of electricity in one direction, but an insulator to current flowing in the opposite direction, is a
    A.   Rheostat
    B.   Saturable reactor
    C.   Capacitor
    D.   Rectifier
    E.   Transducer   1:124

742. All of the following factors affect x-ray beam quality and intensity except
    A.   Tube voltage
    B.   Tube current
    C.   Tube filtration
    D.   Time of exposure
    E.   Target material   1:177

743. The half-value layer of a radiation beam is 3 mm of aluminum. The percentage of the beam that will be transmitted through an aluminum filter 9 mm thick is _____ percent.
    A.   12.5
    B.   25
    C.   33
    D.   50
    E.   75   1:219

744. Ionic bonds are characteristic of which of the following?
    I.   Salts
    II. Acids
    III. Bases
    A.   I
    B.   II
    C.   III
    D.   II, III
    E.   I, II, III   3:14

745. All of the following are properties of magnetic fields except
    A.   All magnetic fields have a north pole
    B.   All magnetic fields have a south pole
    C.   Magnetic fields are displayed by all elements
    D.   Unlike magnetic poles attract each other
    E.   Like magnetic poles repel each other   3:49

746. A pinhole image of an effective focal spot is 7 mm wide. If
     the pinhole was positioned 28 cm from the target and 130 cm
     from the film, the size of the effective focal spot is_____ mm.
     A. 0.5
     B. 1.0
     C. 1.5
     D. 3.0
     E. 4.6   3:111

747. In image intensification, the tendency of straight lines in the
     object to appear as curved lines in the image is called
     A. Penumbra
     B. Vignetting
     C. Modulation transfer
     D. Pincushion distortion
     E. Curvilinear distortion   3:136

748. Photon energy is usually expressed in units of
     A. Half-value layer
     B. KVP
     C. Electron volts
     D. Ergs
     E. Kilocalories   13:15

749. The number of feet in a meter is
     A. 0.305
     B. 0.394
     C. 0.456
     D. 2.54
     E. 3.28   13:334

750. What happens to the incident photon in photoelectric interaction?
     A. It is deflected by an inner orbit electron
     B. It is deflected by an outer orbit electron
     C. It is partially absorbed
     D. It is completely absorbed
     E. It gains energy and proceeds in a different direction 4:78

751. The output voltage from the high voltage transformer in the
     typical x-ray circuit changes polarity _____ times per second.
     A. 15
     B. 30
     C. 60
     D. 120
     E. 240   13:73

752. One pound is the equivalent of _____ kilogram (s).
     A. 0.268
     B. 0.4536
     C. 1.39
     D. 2.2046
     E. 6.1   6:903

For each word or phrase, select the one heading which is most closely related to it. Each heading may be used once, more than once, or not at all.

753. Local deposition of radiation   A. Contrast enhancement
      energy in the irradiated object   B. Absorption
                                             C. Specific ionization
754. Reduction in intensity of the   D. Attenuation
      x-ray beam as it traverses matter   E. Transmutation
                                                                    7:17

755. Characteristics of electromagnetic radiation include
        I. Identical velocity in all materials
       II. The ability to penetrate objects
      III. It travels in straight lines
        A. I
        B. II
        C. III
        D. I, II, III
        E. II, III   7:2

756. X-ray tube current is measured in
        A. Electron volts
        B. Kilovolts
        C. Kilovolts peak
        D. Milliamperes
        E. Brems   7:5

757. Results of keeping the x-ray field as small as possible include
        I. A significant reduction in patient exposure
       II. An improvement in the radiographic image
      III. A pronounced hardening of the x-ray beam
        A. I
        B. II
        C. III
        D. I, II
        E. I, II, III   7:7

758. What is the effect of milliamperage on the x-ray energy spectrum?
        A. An increase in milliamperage produces higher energy photons
        B. An increase in milliamperage produces lower energy photons
        C. An increase in milliamperage produces less ripple in the
            electrical waveform
        D. An increase in milliamperage produces more ripple in the
            electrical waveform
        E. Changes in milliamperage have no effect on the energy
            spectrum   7:10

759. Results of Compton interaction include
        I. The Compton electron receives the total energy of the
            incident photon
       II. A newly created scattered photon moves in a direction
            different from the incident photon
      III. The interaction occurs between an x-ray photon and a
            tightly bound electron
        A. I
        B. II
        C. III
        D. I, III
        E. II, III   7:17

760. The quantity of radiation delivered by an x-ray exposure is a direct function of which of the following?
      I.   Tube current
     II.   Exposure time
    III.   Object-film distance
      A.   I
      B.   I, II
      C.   I, II, III
      D.   II, III
      E.   III   7:77

761. Good conductors of electricity include
      I.   Silver
     II.   Copper
    III.   Aluminum
      A.   I
      B.   I, II
      C.   I, II, III
      D.   II, III
      E.   III   1:41

762. Electrical power may be defined as which of the following?
      I.   The rate of doing work
     II.   The rate of using energy
    III.   The energy per unit time
      A.   I
      B.   I, II
      C.   I, II, III
      D.   II, III
      E.   III   1:66

763. A transformer which increases voltage is a (an)
      A.   Field transformer
      B.   Pole transformer
      C.   Autotransformer
      D.   Step-up transformer
      E.   Step-down transformer   1:107

764. Radiation may be specified by which of the following?
      I.   Frequency
     II.   Wavelength
    III.   Photon energy
      A.   I
      B.   I, II
      C.   I, II, III
      D.   II, III
      E.   III   1:162

765. Effects of scattered radiation in radiography include
      I.   It increases the radiation dose received by the patient
     II.   It increases the radiation dose received by the operator
    III.   It degrades the quality of the radiographic image
      A.   I
      B.   I, II
      C.   I, II, III
      D.   II, III
      E.   III   1:202

766. Elements which contain electrons only in their K shells include
    I.   Hydrogen
    II. Helium
    III. Lithium
    A.   I
    B.   I, II
    C.   I, II, III
    D.   II, III
    E.   II   3:11

767. A series circuit supplied by 100 volts has resistors of 10 ohms, 50 ohms and 40 ohms. The current flowing through the circuit is _____ ampere (s).
    A.   0.1
    B.   1.0
    C.   10
    D.   100
    E.   10,000   3:42

768. The most common device for measuring focal spot size is the
    A.   Wire mesh screen
    B.   Spinning top
    C.   Penetrometer
    D.   Pinhole camera
    E.   Infinite spiral   3:101

769. The brightness gain of an image intensifier is dependent on which of the following?
    I.   Flux gain
    II. Minification gain
    III. Refraction gain
    A.   I
    B.   II
    C.   III
    D.   I, II
    E.   I, II, III   3:132

770. The relationship between power and the area through which energy passes is called
    A.   Amplitude
    B.   Intensity
    C.   Absorption
    D.   Attenuation
    E.   Transmission   13:13

771. The overall sensitivity of an intensified receptor system depends on which of the following?
    I.   The gain or conversion factor of the image tube
    II. The efficiency of the optical system
    III. The sensitivity of the film
    A.   I
    B.   II
    C.   III
    D.   I, II
    E.   I, II, III   13:246

772. The boiling-off of electrons at the x-ray tube filament may be called
     A. Fluorescence
     B. Phosphorescence
     C. Incandescence
     D. Activation
     E. Action-reaction   5:112

For each word or phrase, select the one heading which is most closely related to it. Each heading may be used once, more than once, or not at all.

773. Source of free electrons   A. Anode
                                           B. Cathode
774. Method of accelerating electrons   C. Tube port
                                           D. Tube voltage
775. Material to slow down electrons   E. Focusing cup
                                                           13:59

776. Bremsstrahlung radiation may also be called
       I. General radiation
      II. White radiation
     III. Characteristic radiation
      IV. Particulate radiation
      A. I, II
      B. III, IV
      C. I, II, III
      D. II, III, IV
      E. II, III   7:3

777. All of the following are classified as particulate radiation
     except
      A. Alpha particles
      B. X-rays
      C. Neutrons
      D. Protons
      E. Electrons   7:1

778. The threshold of the ionization effect is about _____ eV.
      A. 1
      B. 5
      C. 10
      D. 100
      E. 1000   7:3

779. An x-ray tube anode must possess which of the following qualities?
       I. A high atomic number
      II. A high melting point
     III. A high rate of heat dissipation
      A. I
      B. II
      C. III
      D. I, II
      E. I, II, III   7:5

780. The photon energy composition of the x-ray beam affects which
of the following?
I. The contrast of the image
II. The exposure to the patient
III. The amount of stray radiation
A. I, II
B. II, III
C. I, III
D. I, II, III
E. II 7:7

781. Which concept is most useful in describing and measuring the
quality of an x-ray beam?
A. Tube current
B. Exposure time
C. Spectral distribution of photons
D. Average photon energy
E. Half-value layer 7:11

782. The energy level at which the Compton effect is essentially
the only process occurring is _____ KeV.
A. 50
B. 60
C. 70
D. 80
E. 120 7:18

783. If an object contains equal numbers of positive and negative
charges, it is said to be
A. Filled
B. Neutral
C. Grounded
D. Fixed
E. Dielectric 1:21

784. Good electrical insulators include
I. Glass
II. Rubber
III. Plastic
A. I, II
B. II, III
C. I, III
D. I, II, III
E. II 1:41

785. The resistance of a conductor increases with
I. Increasing temperature
II. Decreasing temperature
III. Increasing length
IV. Decreasing length
A. I, III
B. II, IV
C. I, IV
D. II, III
E. III 1:73

786. The temperature at which tungsten reaches a point of thermionic
     emission is _____ degrees Celsius.
     A. 100
     B. 212
     C. 1000
     D. 2000
     E. 3176   1:121

787. Results of a photoelectric interaction include
       I. The total energy of the incident photon is absorbed and
           transferred to the electron
      II. The incident photon ceases to exist
     III. The incident photon continues in a different direction as
           a photoelectron
     A. I
     B. II
     C. III
     D. I, II
     E. I, III   7:16

788. Which term best describes the penetrating power of an x-ray
     beam?
     A. Homogeneity
     B. Heterogeneity
     C. Quantity
     D. Quality
     E. Intensity   1:176

789. All of the following may be used to specify the quality of an
     x-ray beam except the
     A. Maximum photon energy
     B. Minimum wavelength
     C. Effective photon energy
     D. Maximum MAS
     E. Half-value layer   1:218

790. The electrons in the outermost shell of an atom are called
     A. Ions
     B. Chemical electrons
     C. Valence electrons
     D. Recombinant electrons
     E. Donors   3:13

791. If the maximum alternating voltage is 170 volts, the RMS voltage
     is _____ volts.
     A. 85
     B. 110
     C. 120
     D. 239.7
     E. 340   3:46

792. Grid-controlled x-ray tubes are typically used for which of the following?
    I.   To obtain short exposure times in angiography
    II. To synchronize exposure in cinefluorography
    III. To produce low energy radiation for mammography
    A. I
    B. II
    C. III
    D. I, II
    E. I, II, III   3:110

793. Most image intensifiers provide brightness gains of
    A. 1 to 10
    B. 10 to 600
    C. 100 to 600
    D. 1000 to 6000
    E. 5000 to 10,000   3:133

For each word or phrase, select the one heading which is most closely related to it. Each heading may be used once, more than once, or not at all.

Prefix	Multiple
794. Mega	A. 10^{-9}
795. Centi	B. 10^{-6}
796. Milli	C. 10^{-3}
	D. 10^{-2}
797. Micro	E. 10^{6} 13:14

798. Possible causes of vignetting in a two-lens optical system include
    I.   The camera lens is mounted too far from the collimator
    II. The camera lens is too large to be contained in the overlap area
    III. The collimator lens is too large to be contained in the overlap area
    A. I
    B. I, II
    C. I, II, III
    D. II, III
    E. III   13:247

This statement refers to the next 2 questions: A transformer with 40 turns on the primary has an input voltage of 100 volts, and an output voltage of 70 kilovolts.

799. The number of turns on the secondary coil is
    A. 280
    B. 2,800
    C. 28,000
    D. 70,000
    E. 130,000   1:108

800. The turns ratio of this transformer is
    A. 1:100
    B. 1:200
    C. 1:700
    D. 1:1000
    E. 1:5000   1:108

Section 5

Radiation Protection and Radiation Biology

801. The SI unit of absorbed dose is equivalent to _____ rad (s).
    A. 1
    B. 10
    C. 100
    D. 1000
    E. 10,000   7:12

802. The value of absorbed dose depends on which of the following?
      I. Beam energy
     II. The type of absorbing medium
    III. Beam current
    A. I, II
    B. II, III
    C. I, III
    D. I, II, III
    E. I   1:208

Refer to the following list for the next 2 questions
      I. Granulocytes
     II. Muscle cells
    III. Nerve cells
     IV. Lymphocytes
      V. Connective tissue cells

803. Which cells are most sensitive to radiation?
    A. I
    B. II
    C. III
    D. IV
    E. V   3:76

804. Which cells are least sensitive to radiation?
    A. I
    B. II
    C. III
    D. IV
    E. V   3:76

805. Photoelectric interaction is most likely to occur when the
    A. Incoming photon energy is at least 1.02 MeV
    B. Electron binding energy is much less than the energy of the
       photon
    C. Electron binding energy is slightly less than the energy
       of the photon
    D. Electron binding energy is more than the energy of the
       photon
    E. Electron is loosely bound to the atom   13:104

806. For radiation protection purposes, the recommended MPD for an
    uncontrolled area is _____ mrem per week.
    A. 0.1
    B. 1
    C. 10
    D. 50
    E. 80   13:297

131

807. For male patients, gonadal shielding should be used for which
      of the following examinations?
        I.   Femur
       II.   Abdomen
      III.   Hip
        A.   I
        B.   II
        C.   III
        D.   I, II
        E.   I, II, III   5:375

808. The product of the absorbed dose and the appropriate modifying
      factor for that particular type of radiation is the
        A.   Dose equivalent
        B.   Quality factor
        C.   Linear energy transfer
        D.   Specific ionization
        E.   Background radiation   12:199

809. In Compton interaction, the angle of ejection of the recoil
      electron is never greater than _____ degrees.
        A.   10
        B.   30
        C.   45
        D.   90
        E.   180   8:33

810. All of the following are radioresistant except
        A.   Tumors of the nerves
        B.   The lining of the gastrointestinal tract
        C.   Malignant melanomas
        D.   Osteogenic sarcomas
        E.   Tumors of the muscles   14:181

811. Exposure of the fetus to radiation prior to the fourth month of
      gestation may result in which of the following?
        I.   Termination of the pregnancy
       II.   Major birth defects
      III.   Increased risk of leukemia
        A.   I, II
        B.   I, III
        C.   II, III
        D.   I, II, III
        E.   III   14:177

812. For the entire gestation period, occupational exposure to the
      pregnant woman shall not exceed _____ rem.
        A.   0.01
        B.   0.05
        C.   0.1
        D.   0.5
        E.   1.0   14:175

813. Information required for calculating the thickness necessary
for a primary barrier includes the
I. Weekly workload of the unit
II. Output
III. Energy of radiation
A. I
B. I, II
C. I, II, III
D. II, III
E. III   14:178

814. For total body radiation, the lethal dose is _____ r.
A. 50
B. 100
C. 200
D. 300
E. 400   14:183

815. Replication of DNA occurs during
A. Interphase
B. Prophase
C. Metaphase
D. Anaphase
E. Telophase   12:39

816. Effects of radiation injury to the cell nucleus include
I. Prompt lysis
II. Accelerated mitosis
III. Formation of giant cells
A. I
B. II
C. III
D. I, III
E. I, II, III   12:63

817. Types of low-LET radiation include
I. Megavoltage x-rays
II. Orthovoltage x-rays
III. Alpha particles
A. I
B. I, II
C. I, II, III
D. II, III
E. II   12:112

818. For radiographic procedures, the number of days included in the
safe period for females who may be pregnant is
A. 5
B. 10
C. 12
D. 14
E. 20   12:157

819. An excess or deficiency of certain chromosomes is called
    A. Euploidy
    B. Haploidy
    C. Diploidy
    D. Aneuploidy
    E. Hypereuploidy   12:188

820. The organogenesis stage in the human embryo is _____ days.
    A. 0 to 10
    B. 11 to 20
    C. 11 to 31
    D. 11 to 41
    E. 20 to 60   12:154

821. Which of the following may occur when a photon produced by
    kilovoltage in the radiography range penetrates an object?
      I. It may interact with the object by the photoelectric process
     II. It may interact with the object by the Compton process
    III. It may penetrate the object without interaction
    A. I
    B. II
    C. III
    D. I, II
    E. I, II, III   7:15

822. A dose rate of 10 mr/hr which continues for 30 minutes will
    provide a total dose of _____ mr.
    A. 0.5
    B. 5.0
    C. 20
    D. 200
    E. 300   1:209

823. All of the following factors influence the radiosensitivity of
    the cell except the
    A. Stage of cell division
    B. Size of the cell
    C. Degree of cellular activity
    D. State of nourishment of the cell
    E. Presence of certain chemicals in the cell or in its
       environment   3:76

824. Coherent scatter may be referred to by all of the following
    terms except _____ scatter.
    A. Compton
    B. Thompson
    C. Rayleigh
    D. Elastic
    E. Classical   13:108

825. In radiation protection, the occupancy factor for controlled
    areas is generally considered to have a value of
    A. 1
    B. 5
    C. 10
    D. 50
    E. 100   13:298

826. The reduction of exposure rate as radiation passes through matter is
    A. Interception
    B. Limitation
    C. Compensation
    D. Attenuation
    E. Transformation
    5:488

827. Lymphocytes arise in all of the following areas <u>except</u> the
    A. Thymus
    B. Liver
    C. Spleen
    D. Lymph nodes
    E. Bone marrow
    12:149

828. Charged particles which are produced in interaction between radiation and matter include
    I. Photoelectrons
    II. Recoil electrons
    III. Electron-positron pairs
    A. I, II
    B. I, III
    C. II, III
    D. I, II, III
    E. I
    8:39

829. In the manufacture of x-ray tubes, the specified maximum safe limit of the housing measured at 1 meter from the target is
    A. 0.1 mr/hr
    B. 1.0 mr/hr
    C. 10 mr/hr
    D. 100 mr/hr
    E. 1 r/hr
    14:177

830. Examples of somatic effects of radiation include
    I. Damage to body tissues and organs
    II. Change in blood counts
    III. Reddening of the skin
    A. I
    B. I, II
    C. I, II, III
    D. II, III
    E. III
    14:172

831. Rules governing radiation exposure to the patient during fluoroscopy include
    I. The tabletop should be no less than 15 inches from the tube
    II. The dose rate to the patient should be less than 10 r/minute
    III. Minimal beam restriction should be used
    A. I
    B. I, II
    C. I, II, III
    D. II, III
    E. III
    14:175

832. In a controlled area where access is limited to occupational personnel, the primary barrier must reduce radiation to what level?
     A. 100 mr/week
     B. 500 mr/week
     C. 1 r/week
     D. 5 r/week
     E. 10 r/week   14:178

833. Terms that are used to describe the length of time that a radionuclide will remain radioactive include
     I. Half-value layer
     II. Half-life
     III. Decay rate
     A. I
     B. I, II
     C. I, II, III
     D. II, III
     E. III   14:189

834. The mitotic spindle is formed during
     A. Telophase
     B. Interphase
     C. Prophase
     D. Metaphase
     E. Anaphase   14:41

835. Matching genes on chromosome pairs are called
     A. Phenotypes
     B. Karyotypes
     C. Somatotypes
     D. Alleles
     E. Dicentrics   14:64

836. Recovery from sublethal radiation injury is called _____ recovery.
     A. Bragg
     B. Marcus
     C. Coutard
     D. Elkind
     E. Fletcher   14:116

837. Radiation effects that can be detected only by statistical methods are _____ effects.
     A. Latent
     B. Somatic
     C. Genetic
     D. Stochastic
     E. Nonstochastic   14:160

838. The dose equivalent in rems is equal to the product of the absorbed dose in rads and the
     A. Exposure in roentgens
     B. Linear energy transfer in microns
     C. Relative biologic effectiveness
     D. Quality factor
     E. F-factor   14:199

839. The device which measures the total exposure during a specific
time period is the _____; the device which allows the instanta-
neous readout of the exposure rate at any time is the _____.
A. Dose rate meter; integrating dosimeter
B. Integrating dosimeter; dose rate meter
C. Film dosimeter; Fricke dosimeter
D. Fricke dosimeter; film dosimeter
E. Scintillation crystal; film dosimeter   7:12

840. The SI unit of absorbed dose is the
A. Curie
B. Becquerel
C. Gray
D. Rad
E. Roentgen   1:208

841. The sensitivity of a cell to radiation depends primarily on
the cell
A. Size
B. Type
C. Contents
D. Location
E. Activity   3:76

842. The process in which a photon transfers all of its energy to an
outer shell electron is
A. Photoelectric interaction
B. Compton scatter
C. Coherent scatter
D. The annihilation reaction
E. Pair production   13:103

843. For radiation protection purposes, the recommended MPD for a
controlled area is _____ mrem per week.
A. 1
B. 10
C. 100
D. 500
E. 800   13:297

844. Primary barriers for a diagnostic x-ray unit are designed to
absorb primary rays produced by a maximum KVP of
A. 100
B. 120
C. 150
D. 180
E. 200   5:367

845. Characteristics of a linear-quadratic dose-response curve include
I. No threshold
II. Linear response at low dose levels
III. Linear response at high dose levels
A. I
B. II
C. III
D. I, II
E. I, III   12:165

846. The interaction which takes place between an x-ray photon and
     a tightly bound electron is
     A. The Compton process
     B. The photoelectric process
     C. The Thomson process
     D. Pair production
     E. Unmodified scatter   8:30

847. All of the following are radiosensitive <u>except</u>
     A. Normal bone marrow
     B. Tumors of the muscles
     C. Tumors of the larynx
     D. Tumors of embryonal cell origin
     E. Tumors arising from blood elements   14:181

848. The amount of leakage radiation from an x-ray tube cannot exceed
     A. One r per hour at 1 foot from the source
     B. One r per hour at 1 meter from the source
     C. 100 mr per hour at 1 foot from the source
     D. 100 mr per hour at 1 meter from the source
     E. 100 mr per hour at the source   14:177

849. The most prevalent methods of radiation monitoring are
     A. Blood counts and film badges
     B. Blood counts and pocket dosimeters
     C. Blood counts and free air ionization chambers
     D. Film badges and pocket dosimeters
     E. Film badges and free air ionization chambers   14:175

850. At what time during pregnancy is the fetus most susceptible
     to somatic injury by radiation?
     A. First trimester
     B. Second trimester
     C. Third trimester
     D. Just prior to delivery
     E. During delivery   14:178

851. Factors that determine the amount of backscatter include
       I. Field size
      II. Beam quality
     III. Tissue thickness
     A. I, II
     B. I, II, III
     C. II, III
     D. I, III
     E. I   14:182

For each word or phrase, select the one heading which is most closely related to it. Each heading may be used once, more than once, or not at all.

         Function   Cellular Structure

852. Metabolic breakdown
                                       A. Golgi apparatus
                                       B. Endoplasmic reticulum
853. Protein synthesis   C. Ribosomes
                                       D. Lysosomes
854. Carbohydrate synthesis   E. Mitochondria

855. Protein digestion   14:38

856. Types of death that irradiated cells may undergo include
     _____ necrosis.
     I.   Coagulation
     II. Solidification
     III. Liquefaction
     A.   I
     B.   II
     C.   III
     D.   I, III
     E.   I, II, III   14:62

857. Factors which may modify radiation damage to cells include
     I.   Physiologic state
     II. Chemical modifiers
     III. Oxygenation
     A.   I, II, III
     B.   I, II
     C.   I
     D.   I, III
     E.   II, III   14:111

858. Which portion of the intestinal tract is a primary site of
     radiation injury?
     A.   The rugae of the stomach
     B.   The haustra of the colon
     C.   The crypt cells of the small intestine
     D.   The cecum
     E.   The sigmoid   14:150

859. Gene mutations in fruitflies due to x-ray exposure were con-
     clusively demonstrated in 1927 by
     A.   Puck and Marcus
     B.   The Curies
     C.   Compton
     D.   Rutherford
     E.   Mueller   14:184

860. The inherent filtration of an x-ray tube includes
     I.   The insulating oil
     II. The tube window
     III. Aluminum sheets
     A.   I
     B.   I, II
     C.   I, II, III
     D.   II, III
     E.   III   7:7

861. The local deposition of the radiation energy in the object being
     irradiated is ____; the reduction in intensity of the x-ray beam
     as it traverses matter is _____.
     A.   Radiation absorbed dose; relative biologic effect
     B.   Relative biologic effect; radiation absorbed dose
     C.   Absorption; attenuation
     D.   Attenuation; absorption
     E.   Subject contrast; radiographic contrast   7:17

862. If a total dose of 45 Gy is required in a time of 15 minutes, the dose rate required is _____ Gy/min.
    A. 3
    B. 5
    C. 15
    D. 60
    E. 675   1:209

863. The response of cells to radiation depends on which of the following?
    I. The type of radiation
    II. The total absorbed dose
    III. The dose per exposure
    IV. The interval between exposures
    A. I, II
    B. I, II, III
    C. I, II, III, IV
    D. I, III, IV
    E. I, IV   3:76

864. Characteristics of a material which affect penetration by x-rays include
    I. Density
    II. Atomic number
    III. Thickness
    A. I
    B. I, II
    C. I, II, III
    D. II, III
    E. III   13:128

865. Functions of the reader unit in thermoluminescence dosimetry include
    I. It heats the TLD material
    II. It measures light emitted during heating
    III. It measures ionization in a light chamber
    A. I
    B. I, II
    C. I, II, III
    D. II, III
    E. III   13:307

866. The minimum dose of low-LET radiation known to induce a human cataract is _____ Gy.
    A. 0.5
    B. 1.0
    C. 1.5
    D. 2.0
    E. 4.5   12:172

For each word or phrase, select the one heading which is most closely related to it. Each heading may be used once, more than once, or not at all.

867. Experiment with rabbit testes
868. HeLa cells
869. Activation of water
870. Oxygen effect

A. Bergonie and Tribondeau
B. Fricke
C. Thoday and Read
D. Puck
E. Marie Curie   12:4

871. Correct statements about the gray as a unit of measurement
     include all of the following except
     A. The gray is a unit of radiation
     B. One gray = 100 rad
     C. The gray is independent of the material irradiated
     D. The gray is independent of the nature of the primary ionizing
        radiation
     E. The gray measures the effect of radiation   8:54

872. Desirable characteristics for all devices that measure radiation
     include
       I. An independent source of energy
      II. Reproducible results
     III. Linear response capability
     A. I
     B. II
     C. III
     D. I, II
     E. I, II, III   14:177

873. Practical methods of radiation protection to be observed by
     persons working with ionizing radiation include all of the
     following except
     A. Proper shielding
     B. Proper beam collimation
     C. Proper distance
     D. Correct time for exposure duration
     E. Consistent use of high MA, low KVP techniques   14:173

874. For radiation protection purposes, which of the following should
     be used by the fluoroscopist?
       I. Small field size
      II. Lead/rubber shields
     III. High MA, low KVP
     A. I
     B. I, II
     C. I, II, III
     D. II, III
     E. III   14:176

875. The recommended thickness of lead for a primary barrier is
     _____ inch.
     A. 1/64
     B. 1/32
     C. 1/16
     D. 1/8
     E. 1/4   14:178

876. The Geiger-Muller counter is most effective in measuring or
     counting which type of radiation?
     A. Alpha
     B. Beta
     C. Gamma
     D. X-ray
     E. Mesons   14:192

877. In the human, the total number of chromosomes at the tetrad
     stage of prophase is
     A. 23
     B. 46
     C. 69
     D. 92
     E. 184   12:41

878. Which cell type is most radiosensitive?
     A. Vegetative intermitotic cells
     B. Differentiating intermitotic cells
     C. Multipotential connective tissue cells
     D. Reverting postmitotic cells
     E. Fixed postmitotic cells   12:76

879. Radiosensitivity of cells increases with an increased con-
     centration of
     A. Oxygen
     B. Nitrogen
     C. Hydrogen
     D. Helium
     E. Carbon   12:122

880. Environmental radiation is typically referred to as _____
     radiation.
     A. External
     B. Internal
     C. Scattered
     D. Secondary
     E. Background   12:200

881. In the International System of Units, the unit of exposure is
     equivalent to _____ roentgen(s).
     A. 1
     B. 226
     C. 498
     D. 2273
     E. 3876   7:11

882. Beam filtration is employed in radiography for what reason?
     A. Biological safety
     B. Improved radiographic quality
     C. Operator safety
     D. Beam hardening
     E. Alteration of beam wavelength   1:197

883. Chromosomal changes that have been observed after irradiation
     include
       I. Chromosomes become sticky, resulting in incomplete separation
          at mitosis
      II. Chromosome separation at anaphase is inhibited, resulting in
          delay of completion of mitosis
     III. Chromosome fragmentation may occur
      IV. Chromosomes may be unequally divided among daughter cells
     A. I, II
     B. I, II, III
     C. I, II, III, IV
     D. II, III, IV
     E. III, IV   3:75

884. The attenuation coefficient depends on which of the following?
     I.   The characteristics of the incident photons
     II. The characteristics of the material through which the
          photons pass
     III. The characteristics of the image receptor.
     A.   I, II
     B.   I, III
     C.   II, III
     D.   I, II, III
     E.   I
                                                        13:102

885. Occupationally exposed persons may receive exposure from which
     of the following sources?
     I.   Primary radiation
     II. Scattered radiation
     III. Leakage radiation
     A.   I, II
     B.   II, III
     C.   I, III
     D.   I, II, III
     E.   II
                                                        13:293

Refer to the following list for the next 3 questions.
     I.   Scintillation counter
     II. Geiger-Muller counter
     III. Ionization chamber
     IV. Pocket ionization chamber
     V.   Film

886. Detectors which are used for surveys only include
     A.   I
     B.   I, II
     C.   I, II, III
     D.   I, II, III, IV
     E.   I, II, III, IV, V
                                                        5:366

887. Detectors which are used for surveys and monitoring include
     A.   I
     B.   I, II
     C.   I, II, III
     D.   I, II, III, IV
     E.   I, II, III, IV, V
                                                        5:366

888. Which detector has a minimum energy measurement of 50 KEV?
     A.   I
     B.   II
     C.   III
     D.   IV
     E.   V
                                                        5:366

889. The observation that radiation was emitted by a uranium mineral
     was made in 1896 by
     A.   The Curies
     B.   Becquerel
     C.   Roentgen
     D.   Crookes
     E.   Fermi
                                                        12:3

890. When a photon is scattered at some angle to its original direction without a change in wavelength, the process is called
    A. The photoelectric effect
    B. Thomson scattering
    C. Compton scattering
    D. Pair production
    E. The annihilation reaction   8:26

891. What is the recommendation for the minimum dose level of radiation?
    A. .01 rem/year
    B. .1 rem/year
    C. 1 rem/year
    D. 1.5 rem/year
    E. No level has been established   14:175

892. Systemic effects of exposure to radiation include all of the following except
    A. Shortened life span
    B. Leukemia
    C. Leukopenia
    D. Anemia
    E. Erythema   14:173

893. The number that relates the extent to which x-rays of a specific energy will be reduced in intensity by a unit thickness of a specific material is the
    A. Half-value layer
    B. Tenth-value layer
    C. Filtration thickness
    D. Shielding requirement
    E. Attenuation coefficient   14:174

894. Any material added to the tube port to attenuate the beam is called
    A. Inherent filtration
    B. Half-value layer
    C. Beam attenuation
    D. Added filtration
    E. Internal filtration   14:178

895. Factors that increase the radiosensitivity of cells include
      I. Oxygen
     II. Temperature
    III. Pressure
     IV. Age
      V. Stress
    A. I, II, III
    B. I, II, III, IV
    C. I, III, IV, V
    D. I, III, IV
    E. I, II, III, IV, V   14:179

896. A photomicrograph that shows the chromosome complement of a
     particular cell arranged according to size is called a
     A.   Helix
     B.   Somatotype
     C.   Genotype
     D.   Karyotype
     E.   Chromograph   12:37

897. The substance that enhances free radical injury to cells is
     A.   Nitrogen
     B.   Oxygen
     C.   Hydrogen
     D.   Carbon
     E.   Helium   12:59

898. Factors which may modify radiation damage to cells include
      I.   Quality of radiation
     II.   Fractionation
    III.   Phase of cell reproduction
     A.   II, III
     B.   I, III
     C.   III
     D.   I, II
     E.   I, II, III   12:111

899. Which type of cell is an apparent exception to the law of
     Bergonie and Tribondeau?
     A.   Erythrocytes
     B.   Lymphocytes
     C.   Platelets
     D.   Oogonia
     E.   Spermatogonia   12:149

900. The greatest amount of evidence exists for induction of which
     type of cancer by low-dose radiation?
     A.   Leukemia
     B.   Thyroid cancer
     C.   Bone cancer
     D.   Breast cancer
     E.   Sarcoma   12:175

901. Important equipment specifications which went into effect under
     the Radiation Control for Health and Safety Act include
      I.   Built-in filtration
     II.   Automatic collimation
    III.   Proportionality between exposure and time
     A.   I
     B.   II
     C.   III
     D.   I, II
     E.   I, II, III   12:212

Refer to this list for the next 3 questions.
I.   Fat
II.   Muscle
III.   Bone
IV.   Water
V.   Air
VI.   Aluminum
VII.   Lead

902. From the smallest to the largest effective atomic number, the correct sequence is
A. I, II, III, IV, V, VI, VII
B. I, IV, II, V, VI, III, VII
C. V, III, I, II, IV, VI, VII
D. V, I, VI, II, IV, III, VII
E. VI, V, I, II, IV, III, VII   7:18

903. Which material has the greatest density?
A. II
B. III
C. IV
D. VI
E. VII   7:18

904. Which material has the least density?
A. I
B. II
C. IV
D. V
E. VI   7:18

905. Methods which may be used as indirect measurements of absorbed dose include all of the following except
A. Ionization of air
B. Fogging of photographic emulsion
C. Beam current measurements
D. Thermoluminescence
E. Fluorescence   1:210

906. Exposure from all of the following must be included in radiation exposure dose limits except
A. Natural background radiation
B. Radionuclides
C. Therapeutic radiation
D. Accidental exposure
E. Radiography   3:83

907. The accepted method for determining whether an x-ray machine contains adequate filtration is to
A. Use a Benoist penetrometer at several KVP settings
B. Measure the HVL of the beam at a specific KVP
C. Assess film density with a densitometer
D. Measure the successive layers of filtration material
E. Determine the photographic effect at all possible KVP settings   13:133

908. Advantages of TLD dosimeters over ionization chambers include
     all of the following <u>except</u>
     A. They can measure a much greater range of dose values
     B. They do not change response with photon energy changes
     C. They are dose-rate independent
     D. They do not have saturation problems
     E. They can collect radiation over a much longer time period
                                                                    13:307

909. The half-value layer for gamma rays from a 1-MeV source is
     represented by which of the following?
     I.   1.2 cm lead
     II.   6.8 cm concrete
     III. 10 cm tissue
     A. I
     B. II
     C. III
     D. I, II
     E. I, II, III   12:221

910. Radiations which are capable of ionizing neutral matter include
     I.   Alpha particles
     II.   Beta particles
     III. Neutrons
     A. I
     B. II
     C. III
     D. I, II
     E. I, II, III   8:10

911. Materials which may be used as filters in a film badge include
     all of the following <u>except</u>
     A. Plastic
     B. Tin
     C. Aluminum
     D. Cadmium
     E. Lead   8:101

912. During fluoroscopy, the greatest amount of scattered radiation
     originates
     A. At the fluoroscopic screen
     B. At the table top
     C. In the patient
     D. In the air space between the patient and the fluoroscopic
         screen
     E. In the tube housing   14:175

913. The amount of radiation that may be absorbed by the body in a
     stated period of time without causing appreciable body injury
     is the
     A. Threshold dose
     B. Maximum permissible dose
     C. Exposure dose
     D. Radiation absorbed dose
     E. Doubling dose   14:173

914. Following radiation exposure to the whole body, the red blood
     cell count remains stable for two weeks, and then declines
     slowly. Reasons for this phenomenon include
     I.   The fact that radiation affects the viability of mature
          cells only
     II. The short life span of mature red blood cells
     III. Mitotic delay in the proliferative cell population
     A. I
     B. II
     C. III
     D. I, II
     E. I, II, III   14:177

915. Criteria for minimizing genetic and somatic dosage by radiation
     include
     I.   Familiarity with exposure sources
     II. An understanding of the effects of exposure
     III. The establishment of effective control programs to keep
          exposures at acceptable levels
     A. I
     B. II
     C. III
     D. I, II
     E. I, II, III   14:178

For each word or phrase, select the one heading which is most closely
related to it. Each heading may be used once, more than once, or not
at all.

916. Radioactivity of uranium   A. L.H. Gray
                                        B. Marie and Pierre Curie
917. Fluorescent ability of x-rays   C. Bergonie and Tribondeau
                                        D. W.C. Roentgen
918. Radium   E. Henri Becquerel

919. Experimental radiobiology   12:3

920. The length of time required for the mitotic process in humans is
     A. 10 minutes
     B. 40 minutes
     C. Two hours
     D. Twenty-four hours
     E. Three days   12:43

921. Which of the following cells are most radioresistant?
     A. Multipotential connective tissue cells
     B. Reverting postmitotic cells
     C. Fixed postmitotic cells
     D. Vegetative intermitotic cells
     E. Differentiating intermitotic cells   12:76

922. Cells that participate in the immune response include
    I.   B-cells
   II.   T-cells
  III.   Macrophages
    A.   I
    B.   I, II
    C.   I, II, III
    D.   II, III
    E.   III   12:131

923. Characteristics of the linear dose-response curve include
    I.   No threshold
   II.   Response proportional to dose
  III.   Nonstochastic effect
    A.   I
    B.   II
    C.   III
    D.   I, II
    E.   I, II, III   12:163

For each word or phrase, select the one heading which is most closely related to it. Each heading may be used once, more than once, or not at all.

Anatomical Area   Quarterly MPD

924. Gonads   A. 1-1/4 rem
                                         B. 5 rem
925. Thyroid   C. 7-1/2 rem
                                         D. 18-3/4 rem
926. Eye lens   E. 25 rem
                                                                   12:208

927. Regulations regarding the total amount of filtration required in the x-ray beam have been written by which of the following?
    I.   National Council on Radiation Protection and Measurements
   II.   International Commission on Radiological Protection
  III.   Bureau of Radiological Health
    A.   I
    B.   II
    C.   III
    D.   I, II
    E.   I, II, III   7:77

928. When secondary radiation is absorbed in tissue, effects may include
    I.   Excitation
   II.   Ionization
  III.   Cleavage of molecular bonds
    A.   I
    B.   I, II
    C.   I, II, III
    D.   II, III
    E.   III   3:74

929. Recommended methods for reducing patient exposure include all of the following <u>except</u>
   A. Gonadal shielding
   B. Filters
   C. Low KVP techniques
   D. Fast film and screens
   E. Field-limiting devices   3:86

930. Fluoroscopic tables should be designed so that the focal spot is at what distance below the table top?
   A. 12 cm
   B. 15 cm
   C. 18 cm
   D. 38 cm
   E. 18 inches   13:289

931. All of the following radiation detecting devices will measure beta, gamma and x-radiation <u>except</u> the
   A. Pocket ionization chamber
   B. Film
   C. Ionization chamber
   D. Geiger-Muller counter
   E. Scintillation counter   5:366

932. A substance that increases the damaging effects of radiation is called a
   A. Radiation protector
   B. Radiation sensitizer
   C. Chemical modifier
   D. Thiophosphate derivative
   E. Sulfhydryl   12:127

For each word or phrase, select the one heading which is most closely related to it. Each heading may be used once, more than once, or not at all.

Evidence or device for determining exposure

933. Integrating dosimeter

934. Erythema production

935. Film dosimeter

936. Destruction of bacteria

937. Fricke dosimeter

938. Thermoluminescent dosimeter

939. Scintillation crystal   7:11

Method

A. Chemical
B. Physicochemical
C. Physical
D. Biological
E. Ionization

940. Three half-value layers would reduce the intensity of a beam of radiation to
     A. 1/4
     B. 1/8
     C. 1/16
     D. 1/32
     E. 1/64   8:22

941. The property of lead that makes it useful for radiation protection is its
     A. Thickness
     B. Low density
     C. Filtration ability
     D. Absorption coefficient
     E. Weight   14:177

942. Local somatic effects of exposure to radiation include all of the following except
     A. Cataract formation
     B. Leukopenia
     C. Hyperkeratosis
     D. Excessive brittleness of fingernails
     E. Erythema   14:173

943. The RBE/QF is 1 for which type of radiation?
     A. Proton
     B. Fast neutron
     C. Slow neutron
     D. Beta
     E. Alpha   14:174

944. The thickness required for a protective barrier depends on which of the following?
      I. The type of area
     II. The amount of added filtration
    III. The amount of collimation
     A. I
     B. II
     C. III
     D. I, II
     E. I, II, III   14:177

945. When is radiation most likely to cause congenital abnormalities?
     A. One to ten days after conception
     B. About four weeks after conception
     C. The second trimester
     D. The third trimester
     E. Just prior to delivery   14:179

946. Correct statements about LET include
      I. It increases with an increase in the charge of the ionizing particle
     II. It increases with an increase in the mass of the ionizing particle
    III. It increases with an increase in the speed of the ionizing particle
     A. I
     B. I, II
     C. I, II, III
     D. II, III
     E. III   12:31

947. Which of the following denotes a positive water ion?
     A. HOH
     B. H_2O
     C. H_2O^+
     D. OH^+
     E. HO_2^+ 12:58

948. Late effects of radiation to the skin include
       I. Alteration in pigment
      II. Atrophy
     III. Telangiectasia
     A. I, II
     B. I, III
     C. II, III
     D. I, II, III
     E. III   12:92

949. Dehydration, drowsiness, lethargy, ataxia and convulsions are symptoms of which radiation syndrome?
     A. Subclinical
     B. Respiratory
     C. Hematopoietic
     D. Gastrointestinal
     E. Central nervous system   12:146

950. Types of cancer that may be induced by low-dose radiation include
       I. Leukemia
      II. Breast cancer
     III. Thyroid cancer
     A. I, II
     B. I, III
     C. I, II, III
     D. II, III
     E. I   12:175

951. All of the following are the responsibility of the Bureau of Radiological Health except
     A. Accreditation of Radiography training programs
     B. Overseeing the field of radioactive materials and nuclear medicine
     C. Establishing manufacturing standards for all x-ray producing electronic equipment
     D. Studying the biologic effects of radiation
     E. Developing programs for training and medical applications
                                                        12:209

952. Materials which are generally used for filters in radiography include
       I. Aluminum
      II. Copper
     III. Tin
     A. I
     B. I, II
     C. I, II, III
     D. I, III
     E. II   7:7

953.   Instruments which are typically used as clinical dosimeters
       include the
       I.   Free air ionization chamber
       II. Thimble chamber
       III. Quartz fiber electrometer
       A.   I
       B.   II
       C.   III
       D.   I, II, III
       E.   II, III   1:211

For each word or phrase, select the one heading which is most closely
related to it. Each heading may be used once, more than once, or
not at all.

        Anatomical region   Maximum quarterly dose
                                       limit in rem
954.   Whole body
                                       A.   1
955.   Gonads   B.   3
                                       C.   5
956.   Eyes   D.   10
                                       E.   25

957.   Red bone marrow

958.   Hands

959.   Forearms   3:83

960.   The amount of scatter produced by an x-ray beam depends on
       which of the following?
       I.   Beam area
       II. Object thickness
       III. MAS
       A.   I
       B.   I, II
       C.   I, II, III
       D.   II, III
       E.   II   13:137

961.   Characteristics of the sigmoid dose-response curve include
       I.   No threshold
       II. Response proportional to dose
       III. Nonstochastic effect
       A.   I
       B.   II
       C.   III
       D.   I, II
       E.   I, II, III   12:165

962.   According to the NCRP, the leakage radiation measured at a
       distance of 1 meter from the source must not exceed
       A.   1 MR/hr
       B.   1 R/hr
       C.   100 MR/hr
       D.   100 R/hr
       E.   500 MR/hr   15:211

963. Women who may be pregnant should receive special attention
     during radiography. Advisable procedures include
      I.   Shielding the pelvis as much as possible
     II.   Limiting the number of exposures
    III.   Using a fast screen-film combination
     A.   I
     B.   II
     C.   III
     D.   I, III
     E.   I, II, III   12:213

964. An example of directly ionizing radiation is _____; an example
     of indirectly ionizing radiation is _____.
     A.   An alpha particle; a beta particle
     B.   A beta particle; an alpha particle
     C.   An alpha particle; a neutron
     D.   A neutron; an alpha particle
     E.   An x-ray; an alpha particle   8:10

965. Somatic effects of radiation include
      I.   Depression of the red blood cell count
     II.   The production of cataracts
    III.   The induction of leukemia
     A.   I
     B.   I, II
     C.   I, II, III
     D.   II, III
     E.   III   8:103

966. The amount of time required to receive a specific amount of
     radiation is called the
     A.   Exposure time
     B.   Linear energy transfer rate
     C.   Time of emission
     D.   Exposure rate
     E.   Exposure dose rate   14:173

967. Which type of radiation has a mass of 1/1837?
     A.   Proton
     B.   X-ray
     C.   Gamma
     D.   Alpha
     E.   Beta   14:174

968. All of the following may be employed for protecting the patient
     from excessive radiation except
     A.   Adequate collimation
     B.   Beam filtration
     C.   High ratio grid
     D.   Fast film and screens
     E.   Optimum KVP   14:177

969. Types of ionization chambers used to measure radiation include the
    I.   Cutie pie
    II. Victoreen meter
  III. Benoist penetrometer
    A. I, II
    B. I, III
    C. II, III
    D. I, II, III
    E. III   14:178

970. The unit of radiation exposure is based on
    A. The amount of reddening of the skin on the forearm
    B. The amount of radiation necessary to produce a noticeable change in the number of white blood cells
    C. Radiation quality x radiation quantity
    D. Ionization in air
    E. The amount of energy transferred to tissue from a beam of radiation   12:11

971. Mitotic changes which appear in cancer cells as compared to normal cells include
    I.   Increased mitotic activity
    II. Unequal division and distribution of chromosomes
  III. Tripolar and multipolar spindles
    A. I
    B. II
    C. III
    D. I, II
    E. I, II, III   12:46

972. Five thousand rads is the equivalent of _____ gray.
    A. 0.05
    B. 0.5
    C. 5
    D. 50
    E. 500   12:86

Refer to the following list for the next question
    I.   Gonads
    II. Skin
  III. Gastrointestinal epithelium
   IV. Lymph nodes
    V. Hematopoietic organs

973. Rank these organs in decreasing order of radiosensitivity
    A. I, II, III, IV, V
    B. II, V, IV, III, I
    C. III, II, V, IV, I
    D. IV, V, I, III, II
    E. V, I, IV, III, II   12:142

974. The linear dose-response curve is used to estimate which of the following
    I.   Radiation-induced genetic damage at low doses
    II. Radiation-induced leukemia at low doses
  III. Radiation-induced breast cancer at low doses
    A. I
    B. II
    C. III
    D. I, II
    E. I, II, III   12:163

For each word or phrase, select the one heading which is most closely related to it. Each heading may be used once, more than once, or not at all.

Anatomical area   Annual MPD

975. Feet   A. 5 rem
                                         B. 15 rem
976. Hands   C. 30 rem
                                         D. 75 rem
977. Whole body   E. 100 rem

978. Thyroid   12:208

979. According to NCRP recommendations, the amount of added filtration that should be used at operating tube voltages below 50 KVP is _____ mm.
A. 0
B. 0.1
C. 0.2
D. 0.5
E. 1.0   7:9

980. If the exposure rate is 1/10 R per hour at one meter from a point source of x-rays, the rate at two meters would be _____ R/hr.
A. 1/40
B. 1/20
C. 1/5
D. 2/5
E. 4/5   7:66

981. The radiation effect which is employed by a scintillation counter to measure radiation dose is the _____ effect.
A. Ionization
B. Chemical
C. Thermoluminescent
D. Biological
E. Fluorescent   1:221

982. The maximum permissible whole body dose of radiation accumulated by a 28-year-old radiation worker is _____ rem.
A. 10
B. 18
C. 28
D. 42
E. 50   3:84

983. In order to reduce patient exposure to the lowest possible level, it is generally desirable to use which type of image receptor?
A. The most sensitive image receptor possible
B. The image receptor system which produces the best image quality
C. The most sensitive image receptor which will give adequate image quality
D. The image receptor system which produces the least amount of quantum mottle
E. The image receptor system which produces the most radiographic contrast   13:286

984. The basic categories of reaction of tissue to radiation include
       I.   Local
      II.   General
     III.   Genetic
      A.   I
      B.   II
      C.   III
      D.   I, II
      E.   I, II, III   5:354

985. For cataract induction in the eye lens, how many times more
     harmful is 1 rad from fast neutrons than 1 rad from x-rays?
      A.   2 times
      B.   3 times
      C.   5 times
      D.   10 times
      E.   20 times   12:199

986. All of the following are classified as heavy charged particles
     except
      A.   Protons
      B.   Deuterons
      C.   Alpha particles
      D.   Beta particles
      E.   Mesons   8:10

987. The recommendation for gonadal dosage per million of population
     for the first thirty years of life is that it not exceed _____
     rems.
      A.   Two million
      B.   Seven million
      C.   Ten million
      D.   Fourteen million
      E.   Seventeen million   14:176

988. For general irradiation of the whole body, critical organs include
       I.   Gonads
      II.   Lens of the eye
     III.   Blood-forming organs
      A.   I
      B.   II
      C.   III
      D.   I, II
      E.   I, II, III   14:173

989. The type of radiation that has a mass of 1 is
      A.   X-ray
      B.   Gamma
      C.   Alpha
      D.   Beta
      E.   Proton   14:174

990. The thickness required for a protective barrier depends on all
      of the following except
      A. The quality of radiation
      B. The distance from the tube to the occupied area
      C. The material of which the barrier is constructed
      D. The degree and nature of the occupancy
      E. The amount of added filtration   14:177

991. As a protective device, doubling the distance from the radiation
      source will have what effect?
      A. The quality of radiation will be reduced to one fourth
      B. The quantity of radiation will be reduced to one fourth
      C. The quality of radiation will be reduced to one half
      D. The quantity of radiation will be reduced to one half
      E. The quality and quantity of radiation will be reduced to
          one half   14:178

992. The average range in air of an alpha particle is
      A. 1 cm.
      B. 1 inch
      C. 10 cm.
      D. 10 inches
      E. Indeterminate   12:30

993. The number of nitrogenous bases available for incorporation
      in DNA is
      A. 1
      B. 2
      C. 3
      D. 4
      E. 8   12:48

994. The radiation dose that will produce sterility in a male is
      _____ Gy.
      A. 0.05
      B. 0.5
      C. 5
      D. 50
      E. 500   12:88

995. Transient, slight depression of the leukocyte count may occur at
      radiation doses of _____ R.
      A. 10
      B. 25
      C. 200
      D. 300
      E. 400   12:143

996. The major late somatic effect of low dose radiation is
      A. Life span shortening
      B. Carcinogenesis
      C. Cataractogenesis
      D. Ankylosing spondylitis
      E. Injury to the embryo or fetus   12:174

997.   All of the following are reasons why aluminum is a desirable
       material for filtration in diagnostic x-ray units except
       A.   It attenuates mainly by the photoelectric process
       B.   It is efficient at low photon energies
       C.   It decreases in attenuating efficiency with increasing
            photon energy
       D.   Modest changes in aluminum filtration can markedly change
            radiographic contrast
       E.   It produces a marked decrease in entrance skin dose   7:19

For each word or phrase, select the one heading which is most closely
related to it. Each heading may be used once, more than once, or
not at all.

      Population group   Annual MPD

998.   Occupational   A.   0.17 rem
                                 B.   0.5 rem
999.   Pregnant women   C.   3 rem
                                 D.   5 rem
1000. General population   E.   8 rem

1001. Limited population   12:209

References

1 - Ball, J.L., and A.D. Moore. Essential Physics For Radiographers. Boston: Blackwell Scientific Publications, 1980.

2 - Bontrager, Kenneth L., and Barry T. Anthony. Textbook of Radiographic Positioning and Related Anatomy. Denver: Multi-Media Publishing, Inc. 1982.

3 - Hendee, William R., Edward L. Chaney, and Raymond P. Rossi. Radiologic Physics, Equipment and Quality Control. Chicago: Year Book Medical Publishers, Inc., 1977.

4 - Hiss, Stephen S. A Study Guide To Understanding Radiography, 2nd ed. Springfield, Illinois: Charles C Thomas, Publisher, 1983.

5 - Hiss, Stephen S. Understanding Radiography, 2nd ed. Springfield, Illinois: Charles C Thomas, Publisher, 1983.

6 - Kreel, Louis. Clark's Positioning In Radiography, 10th ed., 2 volumes. Chicago: Year Book Medical Publishers, Inc., 1979, 1981.

7 - Lamel, David A., et al. The Correlated Lecture Laboratory Series In Diagnostic Radiological Physics. Rockville, Maryland: U.S. Department of Health and Human Services, Food and Drug Administration, Bureau of Radiological Health, 1981.

8 - Lovell, S. An Introduction To Radiation Dosimetry. Cambridge: Cambridge University Press, 1979.

9 - McLemore, Joy M. Quality Assurance In Diagnostic Radiology. Chicago: Year Book Medical Publishers, Inc., 1981.

10 - Myers, Patricia A. An Introduction To Radiographic Technique. New York: Praeger Publishers, 1980.

11 - Paris, Don Q. Craniographic Positioning with Comparison Studies. Philadelphia: F. A. Davis Company, 1983.

12 - Selman, Joseph. Elements of Radiobiology. Springfield, Illinois: Charles C Thomas, Publisher, 1983.

13 - Sprawls, Perry, Jr. The Physical Principles of Diagnostic Radiology. Baltimore: University Park Press, 1977.

14 - Stevens, Matthew, and Robert I. Phillips. Comprehensive Review For The Radiologic Technologist, 4th ed. St. Louis: The C.V. Mosby Company, 1983.

15 - Sweeney, Richard J. Radiographic Artifacts: Their Cause and Control. Philadelphia: J.B. Lippincott Company, 1983.

16 - Torres, Lillian S., and Carol Morrill. Basic Medical Techniques And Patient Care For Radiologic Technologists, 2nd ed. Philadelphia: J.B. Lippincott Company, 1983.

17 - Wicke, Lothar. Atlas of Radiologic Anatomy, 3rd ed. Baltimore: Urban & Schwarzenberg, 1982.

Answers to Section 1

1.	C	51.	E	101.	E	151.	B
2.	B	52.	C	102.	C	152.	B
3.	D	53.	E	103.	B	153.	B
4.	D	54.	E	104.	D	154.	E
5.	C	55.	C	105.	C	155.	A
6.	D	56.	E	106.	C	156.	B
7.	A	57.	B	107.	E	157.	C
8.	A	58.	D	108.	E	158.	B
9.	D	59.	B	109.	E	159.	C
10.	C	60.	E	110.	A	160.	D
11.	B	61.	A	111.	E	161.	E
12.	C	62.	C	112.	B	162.	B
13.	C	63.	C	113.	E	163.	E
14.	C	64.	C	114.	E	164.	C
15.	C	65.	C	115.	A	165.	C
16.	B	66.	B	116.	D	166.	B
17.	D	67.	A	117.	B	167.	C
18.	B	68.	C	118.	E	168.	B
19.	B	69.	C	119.	C	169.	A
20.	D	70.	A	120.	A	170.	C
21.	C	71.	D	121.	D	171.	E
22.	B	72.	B	122.	B	172.	B
23.	D	73.	E	123.	A	173.	E
24.	A	74.	B	124.	D	174.	A
25.	A	75.	B	125.	D	175.	C
26.	B	76.	C	126.	B	176.	B
27.	E	77.	A	127.	A	177.	E
28.	D	78.	D	128.	C	178.	E
29.	B	79.	E	129.	B	179.	B
30.	C	80.	E	130.	D	180.	D
31.	E	81.	C	131.	D	181.	B
32.	C	82.	B	132.	B	182.	E
33.	D	83.	E	133.	C	183.	A
34.	A	84.	D	134.	C	184.	A
35.	B	85.	B	135.	C	185.	D
36.	D	86.	A	136.	C	186.	A
37.	C	87.	C	137.	E	187.	E
38.	D	88.	C	138.	C	188.	B
39.	B	89.	E	139.	C	189.	C
40.	E	90.	C	140.	E	190.	C
41.	B	91.	A	141.	D	191.	B
42.	D	92.	B	142.	D	192.	A
43.	E	93.	A	143.	E	193.	B
44.	D	94.	C	144.	E	194.	D
45.	D	95.	D	145.	C	195.	D
46.	A	96.	B	146.	B	196.	E
47.	E	97.	E	147.	A	197.	E
48.	B	98.	D	148.	D	198.	C
49.	B	99.	B	149.	E	199.	C
50.	B	100.	E	150.	A	200.	B

Answers to Section 2

201.	B	251.	D	301.	C	351.	B
202.	B	252.	B	302.	C	352.	D
203.	E	253.	C	303.	B	353.	C
204.	B	254.	E	304.	A	354.	E
205.	E	255.	B	305.	C	355.	E
206.	B	256.	E	306.	C	356.	D
207.	B	257.	E	307.	A	357.	C
208.	D	258.	C	308.	C	358.	B
209.	E	259.	A	309.	D	359.	D
210.	B	260.	B	310.	C	360.	E
211.	A	261.	D	311.	E	361.	D
212.	C	262.	D	312.	C	362.	A
213.	B	263.	C	313.	E	363.	E
214.	B	264.	C	314.	A	364.	D
215.	E	265.	E	315.	C	365.	C
216.	C	266.	B	316.	D	366.	E
217.	A	267.	D	317.	C	367.	E
218.	A	268.	B	318.	D	368.	D
219.	C	269.	C	319.	E	369.	E
220.	D	270.	D	320.	C	370.	B
221.	E	271.	E	321.	A	371.	D
222.	A	272.	D	322.	C	372.	A
223.	B	273.	B	323.	C	373.	E
224.	D	274.	C	324.	C	374.	E
225.	A	275.	C	325.	C	375.	D
226.	C	276.	B	326.	E	376.	A
227.	B	277.	D	327.	D	377.	A
228.	D	278.	D	328.	D	378.	B
229.	D	279.	A	329.	A	379.	D
230.	E	280.	C	330.	C	380.	E
231.	D	281.	C	331.	B	381.	C
232.	A	282.	B	332.	B	382.	B
233.	C	283.	B	333.	A	383.	C
234.	D	284.	D	334.	D	384.	D
235.	D	285.	C	335.	D	385.	A
236.	D	286.	C	336.	E	386.	E
237.	A	287.	B	337.	E	387.	B
238.	A	288.	D	338.	B	388.	C
239.	B	289.	B	339.	A	389.	A
240.	B	290.	B	340.	E	390.	D
241.	D	291.	D	341.	D	391.	A
242.	C	292.	D	342.	D	392.	C
243.	C	293.	B	343.	D	393.	E
244.	D	294.	A	344.	D	394.	D
245.	A	295.	C	345.	D	395.	B
246.	E	296.	C	346.	E	396.	B
247.	A	297.	B	347.	D	397.	B
248.	C	298.	D	348.	D	398.	C
249.	E	299.	A	349.	B	399.	D
250.	D	300.	B	350.	D	400.	E

Answers to Section 3

401.	D	451.	D	501.	A	551.	A
402.	C	452.	E	502.	C	552.	B
403.	E	453.	B	503.	E	553.	C
404.	D	454.	A	504.	E	554.	C
405.	A	455.	D	505.	E	555.	B
406.	B	456.	D	506.	D	556.	B
407.	B	457.	D	507.	B	557.	D
408.	D	458.	E	508.	D	558.	A
409.	B	459.	A	509.	C	559.	C
410.	E	460.	A	510.	D	560.	D
411.	D	461.	C	511.	E	561.	E
412.	A	462.	B	512.	B	562.	D
413.	C	463.	E	513.	E	563.	B
414.	E	464.	B	514.	C	564.	B
415.	A	465.	C	515.	D	565.	C
416.	C	466.	D	516.	C	566.	A
417.	A	467.	D	517.	C	567.	D
418.	A	468.	B	518.	C	568.	C
419.	C	469.	D	519.	B	569.	C
420.	C	470.	A	520.	E	570.	B
421.	A	471.	E	521.	B	571.	D
422.	D	472.	B	522.	B	572.	B
423.	D	473.	D	523.	D	573.	B
424.	E	474.	A	524.	C	574.	C
425.	C	475.	D	525.	D	575.	E
426.	D	476.	C	526.	B	576.	A
427.	B	477.	A	527.	D	577.	A
428.	B	478.	E	528.	C	578.	D
429.	A	479.	D	529.	B	579.	C
430.	B	480.	B	530.	E	580.	C
431.	D	481.	E	531.	D	581.	E
432.	B	482.	E	532.	A	582.	D
433.	C	483.	D	533.	D	583.	E
434.	E	484.	B	534.	A	584.	A
435.	A	485.	B	535.	B	585.	C
436.	C	486.	C	536.	C	586.	B
437.	B	487.	B	537.	E	587.	C
438.	B	488.	E	538.	C	588.	B
439.	E	489.	D	539.	B	589.	A
440.	A	490.	C	540.	B	590.	E
441.	E	491.	D	541.	C	591.	E
442.	E	492.	B	542.	C	592.	C
443.	D	493.	C	543.	E	593.	A
444.	B	494.	B	544.	B	594.	E
445.	D	495.	D	545.	D	595.	C
446.	D	496.	E	546.	D	596.	C
447.	D	497.	B	547.	C	597.	E
448.	C	498.	E	548.	B	598.	D
449.	E	499.	C	549.	A	599.	E
450.	A	500.	B	550.	A	600.	A

Answers to Section 4

601.	B	651.	E	701.	C	751.	C
602.	A	652.	B	702.	A	752.	B
603.	B	653.	C	703.	D	753.	B
604.	D	654.	B	704.	A	754.	D
605.	A	655.	D	705.	E	755.	E
606.	E	656.	A	706.	B	756.	D
607.	D	657.	D	707.	D	757.	D
608.	B	658.	B	708.	A	758.	E
609.	D	659.	D	709.	A	759.	B
610.	E	660.	B	710.	D	760.	B
611.	B	661.	D	711.	D	761.	C
612.	B	662.	D	712.	B	762.	C
613.	A	663.	D	713.	E	763.	D
614.	D	664.	E	714.	B	764.	C
615.	C	665.	A	715.	E	765.	C
616.	D	666.	B	716.	C	766.	B
617.	D	667.	B	717.	E	767.	B
618.	C	668.	E	718.	A	768.	D
619.	C	669.	A	719.	E	769.	D
620.	C	670.	C	720.	C	770.	B
621.	D	671.	C	721.	C	771.	E
622.	B	672.	D	722.	B	772.	C
623.	E	673.	E	723.	E	773.	B
624.	C	674.	E	724.	D	774.	D
625.	C	675.	B	725.	E	775.	A
626.	D	676.	D	726.	D	776.	A
627.	E	677.	D	727.	B	777.	B
628.	D	678.	B	728.	C	778.	C
629.	E	679.	B	729.	E	779.	E
630.	B	680.	B	730.	A	780.	D
631.	D	681.	B	731.	D	781.	E
632.	B	682.	E	732.	C	782.	D
633.	E	683.	D	733.	C	783.	B
634.	B	684.	D	734.	B	784.	D
635.	C	685.	D	735.	E	785.	A
636.	D	686.	B	736.	A	786.	D
637.	D	687.	A	737.	A	787.	D
638.	E	688.	E	738.	D	788.	D
639.	B	689.	C	739.	E	789.	D
640.	C	690.	D	740.	C	790.	C
641.	A	691.	B	741.	D	791.	C
642.	C	692.	B	742.	D	792.	D
643.	C	693.	D	743.	A	793.	D
644.	D	694.	C	744.	E	794.	E
645.	E	695.	E	745.	C	795.	D
646.	C	696.	D	746.	C	796.	C
647.	D	697.	D	747.	D	797.	B
648.	D	698.	D	748.	C	798.	B
649.	B	699.	A	749.	E	799.	C
650.	D	700.	A	750.	D	800.	C

Answers to Section 5

801.	C	851.	B	901.	E	951.	A
802.	A	852.	E	902.	B	952.	A
803.	D	853.	C	903.	E	953.	E
804.	C	854.	A	904.	D	954.	B
805.	C	855.	D	905.	C	955.	B
806.	C	856.	D	906.	A	956.	B
807.	E	857.	A	907.	B	957.	B
808.	A	858.	C	908.	B	958.	E
809.	D	859.	E	909.	E	959.	D
810.	B	860.	B	910.	E	960.	B
811.	D	861.	C	911.	E	961.	C
812.	D	862.	A	912.	C	962.	C
813.	C	863.	C	913.	B	963.	E
814.	E	864.	C	914.	C	964.	C
815.	A	865.	B	915.	E	965.	C
816.	D	866.	D	916.	E	966.	E
817.	B	867.	A	917.	D	967.	E
818.	B	868.	D	918.	B	968.	C
819.	D	869.	B	919.	C	969.	A
820.	D	870.	C	920.	B	970.	D
821.	E	871.	A	921.	C	971.	E
822.	B	872.	E	922.	C	972.	D
823.	B	873.	E	923.	D	973.	D
824.	A	874.	B	924.	A	974.	E
825.	A	875.	C	925.	C	975.	D
826.	D	876.	B	926.	A	976.	D
827.	B	877.	D	927.	E	977.	A
828.	D	878.	A	928.	C	978.	C
829.	D	879.	A	929.	C	979.	A
830.	C	880.	E	930.	D	980.	A
831.	B	881.	E	931.	A	981.	E
832.	A	882.	A	932.	B	982.	E
833.	D	883.	C	933.	E	983.	C
834.	C	884.	A	934.	D	984.	E
835.	D	885.	D	935.	B	985.	D
836.	D	886.	C	936.	D	986.	D
837.	D	887.	E	937.	A	987.	D
838.	D	888.	D	938.	C	988.	E
839.	B	889.	B	939.	C	989.	E
840.	C	890.	B	940.	B	990.	E
841.	B	891.	E	941.	D	991.	B
842.	A	892.	E	942.	B	992.	A
843.	C	893.	E	943.	D	993.	D
844.	C	894.	D	944.	A	994.	C
845.	D	895.	E	945.	B	995.	B
846.	B	896.	D	946.	B	996.	B
847.	B	897.	B	947.	C	997.	D
848.	D	898.	E	948.	D	998.	D
849.	D	899.	B	949.	E	999.	B
850.	A	900.	A	950.	C	1000.	A
						1001.	B